SOCIAL SKILLS TRAINING FOR PSYCHIATRIC PATIENTS

ROBERT PAUL LIBERMAN

UCLA School of Medicine, Brentwood West Los Angeles VA
Medical Center and Camarillo State Hospital

WILLIAM J. DeRISI

California Department of Mental Health, Sacramento

KIM T. MUESER

Medical College of Pennsylvania at Eastern Pennsylvania
Psychiatric Institute

PERGAMON PRESS

New York • Oxford • Beijing • Frankfurt
São Paulo • Sydney • Tokyo • Toronto

Pergamon Press Offices:

U.S.A.	Pergamon Press, Inc., Maxwell House, Fairview Park, Elmsford, New York 10523, U.S.A.
U.K.	Pergamon Press plc, Headington Hill Hall, Oxford OX3 0BW, England
PEOPLE'S REPUBLIC OF CHINA	Pergamon Press, Qianmen Hotel, Beijing, People's Republic of China
FEDERAL REPUBLIC OF GERMANY	Pergamon Press GmbH, Hammerweg 6, D-6242 Kronberg, Federal Republic of Germany
BRAZIL	Pergamon Editora Ltda, Rua Eça de Queiros, 346, CEP 04011, São Paulo, Brazil
AUSTRALIA	Pergamon Press Australia Pty Ltd., P.O. Box 544, Potts Point, NSW 2011, Australia
JAPAN	Pergamon Press, 8th Floor, Matsuoka Central Building, 1-7-1 Nishishinjuku, Shinjuku-ku, Tokyo 160, Japan
CANADA	Pergamon Press Canada Ltd., Suite 271, 253 College Street, Toronto, Ontario M5T 1R5, Canada

Library of Congress Cataloging in Publication Data

Liberman, Robert Paul, 1937-
    Social skills training for psychiatric patients / Robert Paul Liberman, William J. DeRisi, Kim T. Mueser.
      p.   cm. -- (Psychology practitioners guidebooks)
    Bibliography: p.
    Includes index.
    ISBN 0-08-034695-2:   ISBN 0-08-034694-4 (pbk.)
    1. Psychiatric hospital patients--Rehabilitation. 2. Social skills--Study and teaching. I. Mueser, Kim Tornvall. II. DeRisi, William J. III. Title. IV. Series.
RC439.5.L53   1989
158'.2--dc19   88-28992
                                               CIP

Printed in the United States of America

Coventry University

The paper used in this publication meets the minimum requirements of American National Standard for Information Sciences -- Permanence of Paper for Printed Library Materials, ANSI Z39.48-1984

Dedication

To Janet Brown-Liberman whose personal qualities and skills have made possible the work required to bring this book to life.

and

To the millions of persons with psychiatric disorders who lack personal effectiveness, who have difficulty meeting their social and material needs, and who are acted upon by others rather than take an active part in their lives.

Contents

Foreword

by Ransom J. Arthur, M.D.
Dean, University of Oregon School of Medicine (1978–83)
Professor of Psychiatry, UCLA School of Medicine (1962–78, 1983–88)
Chief of Staff, Brentwood VA Medical Center (1983–88)

We live in an age of enormous neuroscientific advances. Our preliminary understanding of the basic biological mechanisms involved in major mental disorders has been established, although we are merely at the first, rudimentary way station of knowledge in this area. This is also an era replete with psychopharmacological therapies for all manner of disorders construed as nervous or mental.

Similarly, there is a vast body of literature extant dealing with psychodynamics, family interactions, and social and psychological factors affecting serious mental disorders. However, in spite of this plentitude of knowledge, when one turns to the actual care of seriously disabled patients with mental disorders—exemplified, above all, by those suffering with schizophrenia—we encounter a paucity of methods for helping them acquire social and living skills. The learning of these skills, so important for quality of life and community adaptation, has only recently been subsumed within the mainstream of psychiatry.

Whatever the cause of the serious deficits in social and independent living skills that plague psychiatric patients—be it faulty brain functioning, a wretched upbringing, a harsh society, or any combination thereof—the fact is that many chronic mental patients are unable to perform some of the most simple tasks of living. These lacunae can include an absolute or relative inability to initiate conversations, to carry out self-care and grooming, to develop and maintain friendships, to look for a job, and myriad other skills carefully delineated in this volume. The five chapters of the book address the rationale of training in social skills, the means of assessment of such skills, and the methods of training patients in these invaluable assets to successful living in a sometimes implacable milieu.

This work is truly a guidebook—succinct, concrete, clearly written, and unambiguously specific. Based upon learning principles, the text naturally presents a linear and hierarchical exposition. The reader is never in doubt about what steps should follow what step. Each topic is broken down into readily assimilable components. The format, rather like a kit for a ship model, offers the possibility of universality of application of methods for social skills training. Social skills training is coming into use all over the world as a psychiatric technique because the Liberman group at UCLA has fashioned the training methods in such a way that American, German, French, Japanese, Norwegians, or any other national group can rapidly use the training components with their own patients.

Some psychiatrists and other mental health professionals, particularly those steeped in psychodynamics, may find this approach repellent. They may regard it as mechanical, rigid, and overly structured and lacking in all the nuances and subtleties of depth psychology. This criticism ignores the vitality, spontaneity, and directness that one sees in a social skills training group, where patients and therapists are engaged actively in a mutually respectful learning process; moreover, a tour of duty in any mental hospital or community mental health center that serves severely and chronically ill patients will soon convince the observant therapist that, quite apart from drugs and conventional psychotherapy, additional rehabilitation is needed. Patients with a chronic physical handicap such as the poststroke condition often require prolonged physical therapy to regain the maximum functioning possible. In a similar vein, even if, miraculously, the chronic schizophrenic patient lost all trace of a thought disorder and began thinking with absolute lucidity, he might very well not know how to initiate a conversation, or cook a meal, or seek out a job. Rehabilitative training is obligatory if the patient is to have a real chance to make it successfully outside of a protected environment.

Learning these skills is much closer to learning how to fly an airplane or to ice skate than it is to the working-through process of dynamic psychotherapy. Flight training follows a strict syllabus, step by clearly prescribed step. If the trainee successfully masters each step, *Voila!*, the day comes when he or she can fly an airplane. Along the way, the instructor positively reinforces the correct maneuvers of the part of the trainee and tends to extinguish improper actions. The social skills therapist operates in the same mode, reinforcing the patient's gains on the road toward mastery. If social skills training is helpful to patients, it further reinforces the catholicity of approaches that are necessary for the patient to benefit optimally from what healers have to offer. There are no inherent conflicts among drug therapy, psychotherapy, family therapy, and social skills training. Indeed, they are complementary and possibly synergistic. Paradoxically, at the clinical level of actual practice, social skills training is far less mechanical than it seems to be on paper because it involves human beings in a collaborative, constructive, and positive effort aimed toward gaining personal effectiveness and autonomy on the part of the patient.

Professor Liberman and his colleagues have been working productively in the unglamorous and often neglected vineyard of psychiatric rehabilitation for many years. The fruits of their labors are being utilized around the globe. Their lessons carry with them a steady optimism, a sense that every patient can be helped. Even if a cure is not at hand, as it is not in physical disorders such as diabetes and rheumatoid arthritis either, there is no reason for despair. Teaching regressed patients how to make friends is a small but concrete triumph for both patients and therapist and is a blow to therapeutic nihilism. Biological reductionism is often associated with ignoring the quality of life of patients that, in its subterranean form, is endemic in psychiatric circles, especially vis-à-vis chronic patients.

The Liberman group is to be congratulated on yet another excellent contribution to the welfare of the mentally ill, and to the provision of a set of useful tools to the mental health and rehabilitation professions.

Preface

Social skills training, encompassing methods for improving interpersonal relations in activities of daily living, families, jobs, and friendships, has become an innovative and effective avenue for treatment and rehabilitation of a wide variety of psychiatric patients. Building skills in patients with mental disorders is based on the assumption that personal coping and competence can override or buffer the noxious effects of stress and vulnerability in reducing relapses, interrupting chronicity, and improving psychosocial functioning. Because the capacity to deal effectively in a wide range of social and emotional situations provides nonspecific, generic protection from stressful life events and ambient environmental tensions and conflicts, social skills training can be a useful intervention in all psychiatric conditions and in normal individuals and those at risk for mental disorders as well.

As a broad-spectrum behavioral therapy, social skills training is an effective means of teaching patients from varied walks of life and educational backgrounds the emotionally expressive and interpersonal skills necessary for community adaptation. Many of the principles by which learning occurs have been harnessed together to form the procedures of social skills training—social modeling, prompting, shaping, repeated practice, behavioral rehearsal, focused instructions, reinforcement, and homework. The procedures have been arrayed in highly structured and concretely specified fashion, so they are replicable and readily adaptable to many different clinical facilities and settings. The procedures have been described in treatment manuals, enabling research and evaluation to document their efficacy. Social skills training can sometimes effectively serve as the sole treatment for a particular patient or disorder, but more often, it is embedded in a more comprehensive therapeutic program that includes psychoactive medication and other psychosocial services and modalities.

WHO CAN USE THIS GUIDEBOOK?

This guidebook has been written for all disciplines in the mental health, counseling, and rehabilitation professions. It will be useful for highly trained psychiatrists, psychologists, and social workers as well as for paraprofessionals who have only a bachelor's degree or less. No special professional training is necessary for grasping and gaining competence and confidence as a trainer of social skills. Naturally, in-depth experience with assessing and treating psychiatric patients will provide a firm foundation and context for appropriate use of social skills training techniques. To the extent that a clinician "knows" his or her patient—in terms of the limitations and realistic options that a mental disorder poses—the application of social skills training will be properly directed.

Clinicians who can make use of this book include

1. Psychiatrists, psychologists, social workers, nurses, occupational and recreation therapists, rehabilitation counselors, and psychiatric aides and technicians.
2. Pastoral counselors and other clergy who are called upon to assist their parishioners with personal problems.
3. Family physicians who treat large numbers of patients with "functional," psychosomatic, or medical problems that are aggravated by interpersonal stress.
4. Psychotherapists, child care workers, and marriage and family counselors of all persuasions who wish to add an effective technique to their clinical repertoires.
5. Teachers and school counselors who are interested in preventive intervention and who want a technique that can help to improve classroom behavior, teacher-student relationships, and peer relations among students.
6. Personnel officers and business management consultants who can utilize the educative elements of social skills training to improve morale, productivity, and relations among co-workers as well as between supervisors and employees.

There are two types of personal factors that often predict how quickly a person can learn to do social skills training and become proficient in its techniques—basic interpersonal skills and practicality. Because teaching social skills to others requires the trainer to demonstrate these skills himself or herself, basic human skills such as empathy, warmth, spontaneity, sensitivity, genuineness, and a capacity to express all forms of emotions should be part and parcel of the trainer's therapeutic style.

Similarly, a practical and down-to-earth approach to patients, with an active and directive stance, will well endow a clinician intent on using social skills training. These natural, open, and transparent ways of interacting with patients will more often determine the effectiveness of a social skills trainer than will educational and disciplinary background.

The user of this guidebook will be introduced to the rationale for social skills training in Chapter 1, as well as given an overview of what constitutes social skills and their determinants. In Chapter 2, the reader will learn how to evaluate a patient's deficits and needs for specific social skills and how to assist the patient in setting discrete goals for training. With the help of abundant clinical vignettes and verbatim transcripts from actual training sessions, the reader will learn how to conduct social skills training in Chapter 3. Although social skills training can be used in individual and family sessions, efficiency and clinical experience point toward the benefits of the group format; hence, the illustrations in Chapter 3 are taken from a social skills training group.

In Chapter 4, the use of social skills training in developing heterosocial or peer relationship skills is demonstrated, also with ample vignettes and verbatim dialogues from a group for friendship and dating skills. The final chapter highlights some of the problems frequently encountered in social skills training—such as resistance by patients—and how to overcome these problems.

DEVELOPMENT OF SOCIAL SKILLS TRAINING

While social skills training as a therapeutic approach in psychiatric practice was developed and refined by dozens of clinicians who wrote journal articles and books describing their experiences, the methods delineated in this guidebook were first employed by Robert Paul Liberman in 1970 at the Oxnard (California) Mental Health Center. Liberman devised the sequence of steps in the training process and taught the method to the interdisciplinary staff of the center who applied it to the diverse problems presented by outpatients and day hospital patients. The procedures were refined and empirically evaluated by Liberman, William J. DeRisi, and Larry W. King from 1972 through 1975 and then were disseminated in a large-scale nationwide field test in 50 community mental health centers. This field test documented the broad applicability of the procedures in the hands of line-level clinicians working with over a thousand patients.

This successful experience led to the publication of a manual for clinicians, *Personal Effectiveness: Guiding People to Assert Themselves and Improve their Social Skills*, by Liberman, King, DeRisi, and McCann, which sold over 12,000 copies to clinicians who used it in state, VA, and private psychiatric hospitals; institutions for the retarded; mental health clinics and centers; and private offices. The term "personal effectiveness" was chosen because it was easily understood by patients, and it reflected our view that the best indicator of the successful outcome of skills training was not just the improved *quality* of patients' behavior but also the *effect* that this behavior had on his or her social life.

From 1979 to 1981, the techniques comprising social skills training were further developed and elaborated by Charles J. Wallace and Liberman in a controlled clinical trial with schizophrenic patients who were at high risk of relapse. Wallace added provisions for assessing and remediating cognitive deficits of schizophrenic patients in "receiving" and "processing" social information, prior to emitting a response in an interpersonal situation. This innovation added the feature of training patients in *social problem solving* and resulted in generalized improvements in social skills as well as reduced relapse rates. Since 1981, the social skills training techniques have been even more systematically packaged into *modules* by Wallace, Liberman, and their colleagues at the UCLA Clinical Research Center for Schizophrenia and Psychiatric Rehabilitation and the Brentwood VA Medical Center's Rehabilitation Service in Los Angeles. The modular approach to social skills training is exemplified in Chapter 4 and comprises a trainer's manual, patient's workbook, and demonstration videocassette. Experimental studies and national field tests have revealed that patients with severe, long-term mental disorders such as schizophrenia can learn and retain skills taught in modules devoted to teaching medication self-management, symptom self-management, social problem-solving, and recreation for leisure.

This guidebook is aimed at practicing clinicians who are responsible for the care and treatment of psychiatric patients: It is not laced in the theory or research data. To streamline the text as a practical guidebook, we chose to omit references to the professional literature. We are sensitive to the ethical and professional hazards of offering a psychiatric technique without adequate documentation of its safety and efficacy. However, two decades of experimental research, field testing, and program evaluation of social skills training have clearly shown its effectiveness with a diversity of clinical disorders and problems in the hands of hundreds of therapists in many different settings. This body of research is referenced in the Annotated Bibliography located in this guidebook. We have chosen to refer readers to the voluminous literature rather than try to summarize it here to avoid diluting the practical and clinical focus of this guidebook.

GAINING COMPETENCE AS A
SOCIAL SKILLS TRAINER

A conscientious reading and positive response to this guidebook, including completion of the PRACTICE EXERCISES, will prepare clinicians to conduct social skills training with psychiatric patients. The degree of competence and confidence in performing social skills training, however, will depend upon the individual's previous experience with behavior therapy, with using active and directive modes with patients, and with working clinically with psychiatric patients. Novices in the mental health and rehabilitation professions—such as trainees in psychiatry, psychology, counseling, social work, nursing, therapeutic recreation, and occupational therapy—will have the advantage of not having to "unlearn" other modalities and conceptualizations before launching into the active style and behavioral orientation required by social skills training. On the other hand, trainees will lack the experience possessed by their more experienced colleagues in evaluating problems and setting goals with psychiatric patients. While some readers of this guidebook, because of naturally acquired or previously learned skills, will be able to do social skills training with the text as their sole guide, many others will require additional training, hands-on experience, supervision or consultation.

The best way to gain competence is through direct exposure and experience. This can often be arranged by serving as a co-therapist or apprentice to a more experienced and competent colleague who then serves as a role model and instructor. Making sure that you reinforce yourself for your initial steps in applying social skills training is important, so don't choose resistant patients in your fledgling efforts. If the opportunity to learn-by-doing is not available with the tutelage of a more experienced colleague or consultant, it may be worthwhile to attend workshops or even contract with a consultant to provide focused training in your office, clinic, hospital, or center. While some readers of this guidebook, because of naturally acquired or previously learned skills, will be able to do social skills training with the text as their sole guide, many others will require additional training, hands-on experience, supervision, or consultation. We recommend a variety of supplementary learning experiences for neophytes in behavior therapy and social skills training. The following organizations can provide guidance in your becoming a competent social skills trainer, as well as training materials and referrals to consultants and continuing education opportunities:

1. Attendance at the training institutes and workshops offered by the Association for Advancement of Behavior Therapy at its annual meetings. Obtain consultation from experienced behavior therapists and

social skills trainers listed in the AABT Membership Directory. For information, contact

Association for Advancement of Behavior Therapy
15 West 36th St.
New York, New York 10018
(212) 279-7970

2. Use of packaged modules for training a range of social and independent living skills; use of training videos and manuals developed for various mental health and rehabilitation disciplines. Obtain consultation and training workshops from staff of the Clinical Research Center. Available by contacting

Dissemination Coordinator
Camarillo-UCLA Clinical Research Center
Box A
Camarillo, CA 93011
(805) 484-5663

3. Obtain consultation and training from the Center for Rehabilitation Research and Training in Mental Health by contacting

William Anthony, Ph.D.
Center for Rehabilitation Research & Training
Boston University—Sargent College of Allied
   Health Professions
1019 Commonwealth Ave.
Boston, MA 02215
(617) 353-3549

We solicit from readers of this guidebook positive and negative reactions since we plan to update and improve it periodically. We are particularly eager to benefit from clinicians' experiences when attempting to employ the techniques described in the guidebook so that we may establish more specific uses and limitations of social skills training with psychiatric patients. Please write to

Robert Paul Liberman, M.D.
Camarillo-UCLA Clinical Research Center
Box A
Camarillo, CA 93011

Acknowledgments

This guidebook is a distillation of 17 years of experience in developing, evaluating, researching, and refining methods for training psychiatric patients in social and emotional skills. The experience has been accumulated in a variety of clinical facilities and with many different types of patients—at the Oxnard Community Mental Health Center, Camarillo State Hospital, Brentwood VA Medical Center, UCLA Neuropsychiatric Institute & Hospital, and the Eastern Pennsylvania Psychiatric Institute and in private practice.

Many professional colleagues have contributed to the development and validation of the social skills training techniques described in this guidebook, most notably, Charles J. Wallace, Ph.D.; Thad Eckman, Ph.D.; Timothy G. Kuehnel, Ph.D.; Gayla Blackwell, R.N., M.S.W.; Larry W. King, Ph.D.; and Ian R. H. Falloon, M.D. Working with us has been a host of clinicians from the full spectrum of the mental health and rehabilitation disciplines who have carried out social skills training with thousands of patients in research studies and ordinary practice to make the methods worthy of disseminating more widely through this guidebook.

Parts of this guidebook are revisions and updates from the book *Personal Effectiveness: Guiding People to Assert Themselves and Improve Their Social Skills*, which was written by Robert Paul Liberman, Larry W. King, William J. DeRisi, and Michael McCann (Champaign, IL: Research Press, 1975). A professional-quality film and video demonstrating the methods of social skills training, plus a program guide for inservice training or graduate and continuing education make excellent accompaniments to this guidebook for persons wanting to gain competence in doing social skills training—these are available by writing to

Robert Paul Liberman, M.D.
Camarillo-UCLA Research Center
Box A
Camarillo, CA 93011

Chapter 1
Why Teach Social Skills to Psychiatric Patients?

Humans are social, gregarious creatures who need to interact with others to meet their emotional, social, and biological needs. Without the ability to communicate our needs and interests clearly to people who are important to us, our days would be colorless and lonely, devoid of the basic necessities of the warmth, meaning, and nurturance that social contacts and relationships bring to our lives. Such is the plight of psychiatric patients, whose problems in coping with the challenges of daily living stem from their difficulties expressing themselves effectively to their families at home, co-workers and employers at work, clerks in stores, and friends and relatives at social and recreational events.

People with psychiatric disorders such as schizophrenia, depression, and personality disorders usually need assistance and services from caregivers and people in the helping professions. In addition to interacting with family members and friends, these patients must also meet with a variety of people involved in their treatment, including members of inpatient treatment teams, day hospital counselors, board-and-care home operators, other mental health and social service workers, and rehabilitation professionals. Patients who are unable to communicate clearly their feelings and desires to others find enjoyment of life diminished and become more vulnerable to physical or emotional suffering. The cost of not being able to express feelings and have satisfying relationships with other people is high. Psychiatric patients' deficits in social skills can contribute to the worsening of symptoms that, coupled with long-standing functional disabilities, threaten their capacity to care for themselves and cope with daily stressors.

1

SOCIAL SKILLS FOR EFFECTIVE COMMUNICATION

As people go through life, their social skills allow them to pursue their interests, take advantage of opportunities, and live more emotionally rewarding lives. Over time, successes in one's social life gradually shape more effective communication skills, leading to social competence and happiness. Parents, teachers, friends, and media heroes serve as important role models, enabling people to acquire expressive skills through the process of imitation and identification. Skillful interpersonal behavior has naturally rewarding consequences, such as beginning and deepening friendships, reducing life stressors, obtaining material needs, and achieving self-sufficiency. In most cases these rewards are sufficient to motivate people to strengthen and broaden their adaptive social skills.

How are effective social skills normally learned? Appropriate communication and social skills are acquired naturally and spontaneously during socialization, as children mature into adolescence and then adulthood. Social skills are acquired by individuals who are rarely conscious of having learned a complex behavioral repertoire consisting of a combination of small bits of behavior, such as eye contact and hand gestures. Awareness of the learning process involved in acquiring or using social skills ordinarily occurs only when an individual is confronted with a novel or difficult situation that requires new social and emotional responses. For example, people become aware of their assets and limitations in social skills while anticipating an interview for an important job, when called upon to speak at a banquet, or when having to tell someone of the death of a person close to them. To prepare for such challenging and new social situations, people often practice by themselves what they will say, and sometimes rehearse in front of other people as well. One might seek out others who are already experienced at these interpersonal challenges and observe or learn from them. These strategies enable people to experiment with the specific wording they will use in the situation and to anticipate how others might respond to them.

The same methods that people naturally use to learn skills for dealing effectively with new situations are systematically utilized in social skills training with specific patients to teach effective social behaviors: (1) observing another person competently use the skill ("modeling"), (2) practicing the skill in a simulated situation ("behavior rehearsal"), and (3) obtaining feedback and suggestions for improvement from others ("social reinforcement"). Modeling, behavioral rehearsal, and social reinforcement are the learning ingredients that form the backbone of social skills training.

WHAT ARE SOCIAL SKILLS?

In a general sense, social skills are all the behaviors that help us to communicate our emotions and needs accurately and allow us to achieve our interpersonal goals. A variety of specific skills are involved in any successful social encounter. Social interaction can be broken down into a three-stage process that requires a different set of skills at each stage.

The first stage of communication requires *receiving skills*, those skills that are necessary to attend to and perceive accurately the relevant social information contained in situations. Since the appropriateness of our interpersonal behavior is usually situationally specific, choosing the correct social behaviors depends heavily upon accurately recognizing the environmental and interpersonal cues that will guide us to effective responses. Examples of receiving skills include identifying appropriate people with whom to interact, accurately recognizing the feelings and desires that others communicate, hearing correctly what another person has said, and knowing what one's personal goals for an interaction are.

Once a situation has been accurately "sized up" by good receiving skills, we must choose the response that is most likely to be successful in achieving our short- and long-term goals. This stage of communication requires *processing skills*, those steps that are necessary for choosing the most effective skills for the situation. To succeed in an interpersonal encounter, we need to know what we want to achieve and how to best achieve it. Selecting the most effective skills for achieving the goals at hand requires the ability to *problem solve* in an organized, systematic fashion. *Problem solving* involves generating a list of possible solutions (i.e., potentially effective behaviors), evaluating the relative merits of each solution in terms of their anticipated consequences, selecting the best solution or combination of solutions, and deciding how to best put the plan into action. Thus, processing skills primarily allows us to identify the content of what we will say, as well as where and when the interaction will take place.

After accurately perceiving the social information pertinent to the situation (receiving skills) and identifying the necessary skills for the interaction (processing skills), we will have to perform the skills competently to complete the interpersonal exchange successfully. This third stage of communication requires *sending skills*, the actual behaviors involved in the social transaction. Sending skills include both the verbal content or *what* is said, and *how* the message is communicated to others.

Choosing the right words and putting them together into phrases and sentences gives meaning to our interactions with others. But *how* one talks is often as important as, if not more than, what one says. Choosing our words carefully may make us more articulate, but our style of com-

municating quickly, intuitively, and spontaneously engenders the judg-
ments, evaluations, and reactions from others that determine the effectiveness of our social behavior. How one communicates is determined by
the expressive use of nonverbal and paralinguistic skills. Nonverbal behaviors that are important for successful communication include the use
of appropriate facial expressions, gestures, postures, and eye contact,
and interpersonal distance. Key paralinguistic skills include voice volume, fluency and pacing, affect, tone, latency to respond, meshing of
responses in a conversation, and speaking. These nonverbal and paralinguistic components of social behavior are the media that carry a large
part of the meanings and messages of interpersonal encounters.

Unlike sending skills, the skills inherent in the first two stages of
a communication are not overtly and publicly observable behaviors;
rather, good communication requires accurate social perception (receiving skills) and cognitive planning ability (processing skills) before implementing an effective behavioral response (sending skills). Problems in
interpersonal communication among psychiatric patients may reflect
deficits in any one or all of the three stages, as the following vignettes
exemplify.

Carol's inability to deal with constructive criticism from an employer is
due to problems with her receiving, processing, and sending skills. She
is overly sensitive to any criticism and misinterprets criticism as meaning
that she is not liked by her boss (receiving skills). When she is criticized,
she has difficulty thinking what to say (processing skills), such as requesting further clarification or asking for suggestions on how to improve her performance. Instead, she panics and resigns from her job
(sending skills).

Ted's bouts with depression, made worse by alcohol abuse, are related
to his not knowing the sending skills to resist invitations to drink with
acquaintances. He frequently fights with others because of deficits in
receiving and processing skills. He misreads people as being hostile to
him (receiving skills) and can only think of aggressive responses to cope
with the perceived conflict (processing skills).

Karen has difficulty asking her husband to help her with their children, since she inaccurately anticipates that he will reject her request
(processing skills). Her meek and tentative manner when speaking to
her children often results in their ignoring her, suggesting that by improving her sending skills, she could gain stature in her family.

Allen's avoidance of social interactions reflects his trouble identifying
suitable people and situations in which to initiate conversations (receiving skills). When he interacts with others, he sometimes talks about his

delusions, which frightens other people (processing skills). He speaks in a halting, low monotone with poor eye contact and an absence of gestures and body language, so that people find him uninteresting (sending skills).

Tom is fearful of strangers since he has poor receiving skills. He inaccurately perceives criticism and other negative emotions in the faces and speech of strangers. When he does interact with others, he has trouble thinking of what to say (processing skills).

Elaine's inaccurate processing skills are partly responsible for her troubled relationship with her husband. She assumes that if she communicates a negative feeling to him, he will be angered and might possibly desert her. Actually, such an open expression of feelings would improve their marriage, providing each of them with much needed feedback about how their behavior affects one another.

Jack frequently makes inappropriate statements to others, reflecting his poor processing skills in identifying and selecting suitable topics for conversations. His attentional problems indicate improvements in receiving skills, since he has difficulty following what others say when talking with them.

Samuel has problems with processing and sending skills. When Sam and his parents disagree about something, he is unable to think of a specific goal and generate effective solutions for accomplishing it (processing skills). When Sam becomes frustrated, he shouts at his parents rather than constructively expressing his unpleasant feelings to them (sending skills).

Jane needs help improving her sending skills. As she rehearses verbal, nonverbal, and paralinguistic skills for conveying her interest in dates, she will become more comfortable in these situations and less likely to be at a loss for words.

Albert's difficulty initiating conversations results from deficits in his nonverbal and paralinguistic sending skills, which communicate disinterest and fear instead of friendliness and enthusiasm.

Paul's shyness reflects deficits in all three skill areas. He misinterprets others' communication to him as signifying their dislike and disdain of him (receiving skills). He is unable to plan effectively what he wants to say to others, such as requesting help from co-workers about how to assemble an instrument at his sheltered workshop (processing skills). His style of communication is muted, flat, and nonexpressive (sending skills).

Susan's propensity toward self-injurious and attention-seeking behavior reflects her deficits in receiving and processing skills. She inaccurately perceives others as rejecting her. Rather than directly expressing her concerns and checking out the other person's feelings, she deprecates and hurts herself in despair, thereby pressuring others to intervene and rescue her.

The assertive and socially skilled person takes an active part in his or her work and social life, choosing and achieving goals without taking advantage of others. Therapists and counselors often incorrectly assume that their patients *know how to express* their positive and negative emotions and need only to understand *why* they fail in self-expression. This is often a false assumption, since many people simply do not have the appropriate self-assertive responses in their repertoires and need to be concretely taught *how* to express their feelings.

WHY DO PATIENTS LACK SOCIAL SKILLS?

Psychiatric patients have difficulty expressing a wide range of emotions, including feelings such as closeness and affection, anger and annoyance, joy and happiness, sadness and grief, confidence, and interest and concern for others. Four factors can account for the problems patients experience in communicating their feelings to others:

1. Some people have never learned to express these emotions in the first place because they were not exposed to appropriate role models while growing up with their families or among their friends. Lack of exposure, and opportunities to learn are often compounded by brain neurochemical deficiencies associated with chronic schizophrenia or severe depressive illnesses that may impede learning even when adequate role models are available.

2. The onset of psychiatric illness is often accompanied by and reflected in a severe deterioration in patients' social functioning. The loss of social competence is so cardinal to the development of an illness that some disorders, such as schizophrenia, can only be diagnosed with the *Diagnostic and Statistical Manual of Mental Disorders, Third Edition* (DSM-III) when the characteristic symptoms are accompanied by a decline in social functioning. Furthermore, without social rehabilitation patients usually continue to exhibit poor social competence long after more dramatic symptoms of their illness such as mood disturbances, delusions, or hallucinations have been improved.

3. Environmental stressors such as personal traumas and losses, or sudden changes in one's social world often impair cognitive processing and lead to anxiety or depression which, in turn, interfere with one's spontaneity in social situations. The result is that patients' emotional and interpersonal reactivity is inhibited, preventing them from being socially effective and attaining their personal goals. As stressors inter-

fere with the social functioning and goal attainment of patients, a vicious cycle may develop in which poor skills invite further stressors, which, in turn, further impede social performance.

4. A patient's social environment can change so that social skills that were once supported and reinforced by co-workers, friends, or family members become ignored and fall into disuse, rendering the person powerless to employ these behaviors when an appropriate situation arises. This deterioration in social skills is common in environments where chronic psychiatric patients often reside and is characterized by pronounced social isolation, inadequate social stimulation, and lack of interpersonal resources. Impoverished social settings populated by psychiatric patients include the back wards of state mental hospitals, inner-city streets where patients are "dumped" following brief hospital treatment of their acute symptoms, nursing homes, board-and-care homes, and day treatment centers, all of which are characterized by poor staff-to-patient ratios and a lack of structured programming.

When patients are unable to express themselves clearly, their ability to maintain interpersonal relationships and achieve a satisfactory quality of life is threatened: Poor expressiveness accompanies illness episodes such as during a relapse of depression or schizophrenia. Interpersonal communication is misguided also during the excitement, aggression, or the persistent elation of mania, when patients express their feelings in an overly intense, inappropriate manner. Psychiatric patients, whose problems are compounded by deficient or maladaptive social and emotional expression, often seek help from professionals who are not proficient in providing social skills training. The staff of human service agencies, psychiatric hospitals, day treatment centers, and community mental health centers and the clergy and the police have rarely been exposed to the methods of social skills training. At other times, patients may languish in social isolation, or family members may live in dread of their erratic outbursts, unaware that the methods for improving these behaviors may be available through social skills training.

For example, consider the predicaments of the following psychiatric patients:

Problem Areas	Social Skills Deficits
Carol has schizophrenia and lives with her parents. She has failed numerous times on jobs. She spends much of her time sleeping, to the annoyance of her family.	She has difficulty accepting criticism from employers and is anxious about failing on another job. She avoids her parents since they pressure her to spend more time finding a job.

Ted, with a borderline personality disorder, is prone to drinking too much and getting into fights at bars. He has stormy relationships with others and has trouble maintaining friendships. He has trouble saying "no" to alcohol and tends to misinterpret others' comments insults to him, provoking him to verbal and physical abuse.

Karen has a major depressive disorder that has limited her ability to fulfill her role as a mother and a wife. Even when receiving medication, she feels uncomfortable interacting with others and rarely leaves her home. Her husband has taken over most tasks outside of the home such as shopping and is resentful about this. She does not speak assertively to her children, nor does she request her husband's help with the children when she needs it. She does not know what to say to others and speaks in a monotonous, depressed tone of voice.

Allen has chronic schizophrenia, characterized by occasional auditory hallucinations and delusions and severe social withdrawal. He lives in a board-and-care home but has no friends. His only social support outside of the staff are his parents, whom he annoys by calling many times daily. His disturbances in thinking interfere with finding appropriate topics for conversations with others. His poor communication skills make all social interactions stressful, leading to his avoidance of social situations.

Tom, a schizoaffective patient who lives with his grandmother, has no friends. He spends most of his time in his room listening to music and abuses any drugs he can obtain. He is fearful of people and withdrawn and only talks with his grandmother and caseworker. His abuse of drugs temporarily improves his mood, but also worsens his paranoid thinking and has precipitated several relapses.

Elaine has a dependent personality disorder. She has problems with her marriage and feels unsupported by her husband. She is afraid her husband will reject her if she expresses a negative feeling to him, so instead, she avoids him and withdraws when she is angry.

Jack has a schizotypal personality disorder. He has difficulty making friends and getting along with his family members.	His attention frequently wanders, and he says off-the-wall things. When speaking with others, he fails to acknowledge what they have to say.
Samuel has a manic-depressive illness and lives with his parents. He often has heated arguments with them over household chores.	He and his parents have difficulty agreeing on what the problem is, and he quickly becomes angry and yells at them.
Jane is a college student who has concerns about dating men, but wants to have more intimacy in her life.	She feel anxious with men and "freezes" without knowing how to respond to conversation and affection.
Albert has a schizoid personality disorder, and has come to his clergyman because he is isolated and lonely.	He has trouble conversing with co-workers. When he talks, he speaks quietly in a monotone, and avoids eye contact with the other person.
Paul has schizophrenia and moderate mental retardation. He feels discouraged because he has a very low work rate at the sheltered workshop he attends.	He is shy and unsure of how to ask another client or a supervisor to assist him in improving his job performance.
Susan has a cyclothymic disorder and lives in her own apartment. She has made many suicide attempts and constantly seeks reassurances from other people.	When she feels angry or rejected by others, she seeks negative attention by hurting herself rather than communicating these feelings directly to others.

Therapists can help patients like these overcome common life problems by teaching them how to communicate their emotions and desires more effectively to others. Social skills are the behaviors necessary to overcome these obstacles and achieve personal goals through rewarding interactions with others. Social skills training is the method by which patients can be taught to expand their behavioral repertoires and succeed in social situations where they have previously failed.

Whether patients have social deficits because they never learned the necessary skills when growing up, or whether they learned the skills and later lost them due to their illness and lack of practice, social skills training can improve their functioning and quality of life. Previously competent patients, whose skills have become dormant, can be re-motivated to begin using their social skills again through the instigation, rehearsal, feedback, and "real-world" assignments that are fundamental to social skills training.

Severe psychiatric illnesses such as schizophrenia, manic-depression, and some personality disorders are generally assumed to be biological in origin, even though many of the repercussions of these illnesses are social in nature. How can social skills training, a treatment approach that focuses on teaching social behavior, have an impact and influence on the course of a primarily biological illness? The stress-vulnerability-coping skills model of mental illness provides a useful framework for under-standing the role of social interventions in treating psychiatric illnesses.

STRESS-VULNERABILITY-COPING SKILLS MODEL

The symptoms of most psychiatric illnesses, such as depression and schizophrenia, are believed to be the consequence of two combined in-fluences: psychobiological vulnerability and environmental stress. A person who has the vulnerability to a psychiatric illness has the propen-sity to develop symptoms of the illness under certain conditions. This psychobiological vulnerability is determined mainly by genetic and de-velopmental factors, although drug and alcohol abuse can also influence it. The specific indicators of vulnerability are only beginning to be stud-ied and identified. For example, in those individuals suffering from schizophrenia, vulnerability may be reflected in abnormalities of infor-mation processing as well as in the number of first-degree relatives with the illness.

Stressors are events or contingencies in the environment that have a negative effect on the person and require adaptation, such as life events or an emotionally charged home environment. Not only is too much stimulation, especially when colored with negative affect, harmful to patients saddled with a vulnerability to mental illness, but an *absence* of stimulation can also worsen the course of the illness. Lack of structure or an impoverished social environment, such as is present in some back wards of state hospitals and inadequate living facilities in the commu-nity, can be as stressful as an overstimulating environment and can lead to symptomatic behaviors and social withdrawal.

Social support can reduce the noxious effects of stress on vulnerability by either reducing stress itself or helping to minimize its negative effects on the patient. The greater a patient's vulnerability to the illness, the less stress he or she can be exposed to before developing or worsening his or her psychiatric symptoms. This means that some patients are so vulnerable that they can be continually symptomatic even without being exposed to identifiable stressors.

The effects of environmental stressors on vulnerability are also influenced by the patient's coping skills. Coping skills enable the person either to remove the source of the stress or to minimize its negative impact. Social skills, as defined earlier, are the skills necessary for achieving social, emotional, or instrumental goals, including the ability to manage stress effectively. Thus, coping skills are a subset of social skills that enable a patient to achieve the goals of stress management.

Coping skills or *social skills* are the actual behaviors involved in successful social interactions, including accurate social perception (receiving skills), selecting suitable responses for achieving the goal of interaction (processing skills), and the verbal, nonverbal, and paralinguistic behaviors performed in the encounter. While social skills are the specific behaviors in a patient's repertoire, *social competence* is determined by the impact of the individual's use of skills on the social environment. When social skills are used appropriately in a receptive environment and key personal goals are achieved, the result is social competence, which is the aim of social skills training.

Thus, proficient social skills play a crucial role in enabling patients to remain symptom-free or, with a minimum of symptoms, to lower their risk of symptomatic relapses, and to improve their social functioning. Figures 1-1a, b, and c (p. 13) illustrate the interactions between vulnerability and stress, on the one hand, and medication, social support, and social skill on the other hand in determining a patient's adjustment. Of course, since vulnerability and stressful experiences vary from person to person, some patients will tend to have more symptoms than others, even when they are equally socially skilled. However, teaching social skills to even highly vulnerable patients can nevertheless minimize symptom exacerbations. Thus, enhancing social skills is critical to improving the prognosis of patients with psychiatric illnesses.

HOW TO TRAIN PEOPLE
TO USE SOCIAL SKILLS

In helping individuals to reach out effectively for human contact, obtain their personal needs, and express their feelings, social skills training incorporates well-documented learning strategies that are used in teaching many other human skills. In such training the therapist does the following:

- Breaks the desired behaviors into specific, concrete, manageable steps or building blocks.
- Assesses the individual's assets and deficits in receiving, processing, and sending skills.
- Identifies and restructures the patient's maladaptive cognitions that set negative expectations and impair effective social performance, such as overgeneralizing, jumping to conclusions, catastrophizing, and being self-deprecating.
- Gives clear instructions and prompts for the desired behavior, repeating them as necessary to guide the patient successfully through a rehearsal.
- Has the patient review short- and long-term goals for the situation, and identifies behaviors that may attain these goals.
- Encourages the patient to rehearse the skills under direct supervision.
- Gets the patient to judge the other person's needs, rights, and emotions in the situation.
- Elicits the patient's self-evaluation of effectiveness in achieving the goals.
- Exposes the patient to role models who can demonstrate more appropriate ways of communicating.
- Gives positive feedback and suggestions for improvement, shaping the patient into gradually better ways of communicating step by step.
- Provides explicit "homework" assignments for graded practice in real-life between training sessions.
- Rewards successful approximations of the desired behaviors outside of the session with approval and praise.

These strategies that form the basic sequence of social skills training harness basic principles of human learning. *Positive expectations* are set by correcting false assumptions and negative self-talk. Behavior change is accomplished through a combination of didactic presentation of information, *observational learning* from role models, prompting specific behaviors, and *positive reinforcement* of successive approximations toward desired behavioral goals. The transfer or generalization of skills learned in one environment to another is programmed through homework assignments and practice in real-life situations. Inappropriate or maladaptive behaviors are *extinguished* or reduced by either ignoring them or teaching alternative skills that are incompatible with them.

Once behavior changes have been effected, they are maintained by the naturally occurring social reinforcers present in the environment, providing that the person lives in a sufficiently rewarding milieu.

GOOD ADJUSTMENT

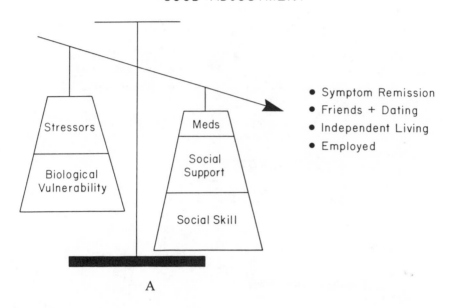

- Symptom Remission
- Friends + Dating
- Independent Living
- Employed

A

MODERATE ADJUSTMENT

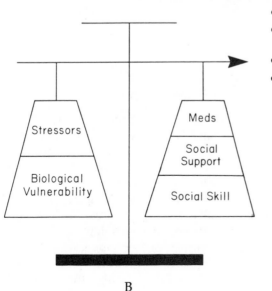

- Symptom Stabilization
- Day Treatment or
  Social Club Attendance
- Half Way House
- Transitional Employment
  or Sheltered Workshop

B

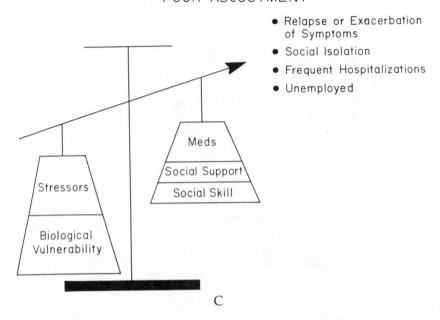

POOR ADJUSTMENT

- Relapse or Exacerbation of Symptoms
- Social Isolation
- Frequent Hospitalizations
- Unemployed

C

FIGURES 1-1a, b, and c illustrate how the balance between psychiatric illness risk factors (biological vulnerability and stress) and protective factors (medication, social support, and social skill) determine the symptom impairments and social adjustment of patients. As patients' social skills and social support increase, their functioning improves, and they require less medication to counterbalance their stress and vulnerability to the illness. Adjustment is divided into four domains of functioning: symptomatology, social activity, independent living skills, and vocational adjustment.

WHAT ARE THE GOALS OF SOCIAL SKILLS TRAINING?

Psychiatric patients can be taught to initiate, maintain, and end conversations with relatives, friends, and strangers. Basic conversational skills can be taught systematically to patients who are shy and withdrawn and who often complain, "I don't even know what to say." They can practice the rudiments of effective conversational skills such as eye contact, adequate voice volume and intonation, proper pacing and fluency of speech, and demonstrative use of gestures and facial expressions. Another important component in sustaining human interaction is giving and asking for information and opinions. Through the use of these skills, patients can learn how to start new relationships, deepen existing ones, and succeed in dating. In Chapter 4, we present detailed descriptions of a social skills training program designed to teach friendship and dating skills to psychiatric patients.

Preparing for job interviews, an important survival skill in community adjustment, is another major goal of social skills training with many patients. Patients can be taught skills to manage their own medication better, to become more informed consumers of drug therapy, and to deal with such problems as calling a doctor to discuss medication side effects. Learning to give and accept criticism is a skill often taught. Standing up for one's rights, the conventional meaning of assertiveness, is important for patients to learn, especially in advocating for their own needs from social service and mental health agencies.

A wide range of patients and their problems have responded favorably to social skills training, as exemplified by a

- chronic schizophrenic man with residual psychotic symptoms who had no friends and only interacted with his family and board-and-care operators.
- 27-year-old man with a borderline personality disorder who frequently abused alcohol, got into fights, and was unable to keep friends.
- 27-year-old woman with schizophrenia who avoided other people and had a history of being fired from or quitting many jobs.
- depressed mother of two children who felt overburdened by child-rearing responsibilities, but who was afraid to ask her husband to help discipline and manage their young children.
- autistic adult with good independent and vocational skills, but who had difficulty relating to other people and accepting criticism.
- middle-aged woman with a substance abuse disorder who was afraid to ask her landlord to make repairs.
- 30-year-old schizoaffective patient who avoided all social contact.
- patient with a dysthymic disorder and an intermittent explosive disorder whose job was in jeopardy due to outbursts of anger.
- 33-year-old schizophrenic man who had difficulty expressing positive feelings to his wife.
- 29-year-old wife who was chronically depressed and who expressed resentment to her husband by sulking.
- man with alcoholism who was unable to stand up to his boss's unfair criticism.
- drug abuser who was unable to express himself and reject overtures to use drugs and who seemed disinterested in other people.
- 50-year-old manic-depressive whom people avoided interacting with because he spoke too quickly.

- 35-year-old woman with a narcissistic personality disorder who alienated people by revealing too much about herself early in conversations.
- 24-year-old retarded woman with an atypical psychosis who lived with her parents and had frequent temper outbursts.

THE EFFICACY OF
SOCIAL SKILLS TRAINING

Controlled clinical research has demonstrated that social skills training can be effective both in enhancing the social competence of patients and in reducing their vulnerability to debilitating psychiatric symptoms, such as depression, delusions, hallucinations, and problems with impulse control. Several studies have found that social skills training significantly reduces symptoms and the risk for relapse in both schizophrenic inpatients and outpatients. Similarly, schizophrenic patients who received social skills training while participating in a day treatment program experienced more durable reductions in symptoms than did patients in day treatment with no skills training.

Social skills training also alleviates depression in unmedicated depressed outpatients. The efficacy of skills training with outpatients with major depression is equal to that of antidepressant medications with this population, and is associated with a substantially lower rate of dropout from treatment. Social skills training has also been found to be a useful adjunct to the vocational rehabilitation of chronic psychiatric patients, regardless of their specific diagnoses. When skills training is combined with other components of effective vocational rehabilitation, such as vocational training and "job clubs" to facilitate successful job finding, patients are better able to reintegrate into the community, economically support themselves, and achieve greater self-sufficiency. The Annotated Bibliography for this guidebook lists publications that contain research and clinical reports of social skills training for different problem areas and patient populations.

SOCIAL SKILLS AND
PSYCHIATRIC PATIENTS

Psychiatric patients need to be taught more adaptive social skills to improve the quality of their lives and to minimize the adverse effects of their illnesses. While social skills training can be helpful to psychiatric patients with even less disabling disorders, many patients with serious and long-term illnesses have a dire need for skills training. Chronically ill patients often have pervasive social deficits that stigmatize them in the community, leading to social rejection and a lack of social support. These patients typically live in substandard housing, are unemployed and unstimulated, and are doomed to a life of social isolation by their inability to create and strengthen social supports that are responsive to their needs.

Social skills training can improve the social adjustment and capacity for independent living of seriously disabled patients by equipping them with the interpersonal behaviors necessary to establish and maintain relationships and the skills to obtain important material needs. As patients' interpersonal skills develop, they are able to strengthen and expand their social networks, which may help to buffer the negative effects of life events and stressors on the patient.

The social skills of patients are an accurate reflection of their social functioning and well-being. These skills also have a direct and reciprocal impact on the severity of their psychiatric symptoms and the likelihood of symptomatic relapses. Symptomatic patients tend to have inadequate social functioning. Through a corollary mechanism, poor premorbid and current social adjustment in psychiatric patients is predictive of negative long-term outcomes, with fewer symptom remissions and more exacerbations and rehospitalizations. The influence of patients' assets in social skills on creating a more benign course of the illness underscores the roll of social skills training as a clinical treatment method that can ameliorate psychopathology as well as facilitate social functioning.

In addition to improving the ability of patients to achieve their personal goals and secure a better quality of life, social skills training can also provide them with the skills to reduce or avoid stressful situations that may provoke a symptom exacerbation. For example, relatives of psychiatric patients may become understandably exasperated by patients' extreme social withdrawal, lack of activity, and apathy, leading them to criticize or be oversolicitous with the patient. These intrusive communication styles, termed high "expressed emotions," can put a vulnerable depressed or schizophrenic patient at a higher risk for relapse. Social skills training can enable patients and relatives alike to learn the skills necessary to recognize and defuse conflict situations, thereby reducing stress on themselves. Furthermore, as patients develop better social skills and become more active, their deficit and negative symptoms improve. They spend more time outside their homes with other people, thus reducing the stress and emotional burden of caregiving on their family members, freeing patient and relatives for more positive social interactions.

Effective social and problem-solving skills lead to interpersonal relationships that facilitate insight and reality testing for patients prone to disordered thinking. As patients gain social approval and begin to integrate themselves into a community, they are exposed to additional learning opportunities through being able to observe others model appropriate social skills. The relationships that patients develop may further improve their adjustment by helping them to set realistic expectations for performance and providing a change to ventilate and express deeply held and often suppressed feelings. Social relationships developed through social skills training can also enable patients to solve their problems better since "two heads are better than one." Relationships with others also provide additional opportunities for patients to monitor the presence and severity of their symptoms. This can lead to earlier recognition of the signs of impending relapse and earlier intervention that can avert a full-blown relapse. The spectrum of reasons for treating psychiatric patients with social skills training are summarized in Table 1-1.

HISTORICAL DEVELOPMENT OF SOCIAL SKILLS TRAINING

Methods for systematically teaching people to improve their social and emotional responsiveness first appeared in the work of Andrew Salter over 35 years ago. In Salter's 1949 book, *Conditioned Reflex Therapy*, he described techniques for facilitating self-expression of neurotic psy-

Table 1-1. Rationale for Social Skills Training

Patients have the following multiple social deficits:
    Poor premorbid and current social functioning
    Negative and deficit symptoms
    Ineffective problem-solving skills
    Cognitive impairments
    Poor quality of life

The following social and environmental stressors worsen the symptoms:
    Lack of social support
    Negative effects of high expressed emotion from family or others
    Life events
    Lack of meaningful structure and social stimulation
    Impoverished living conditions

Social relationships provide the following benefits:
    Social approval and integration
    Material support
    Reality testing and insight
    Realistic expectations for performance
    Modeling
    Symptom monitoring
    Problem solving
    Empathy and ventilation

chiatric patients, which he believed would help them to overcome their anxiety, depression, and other dysphoria. Three decades ago, Wolpe (1958) showed in his pioneering book, *Psychotherapy by Reciprocal Inhibition*, that patients could overcome their social fears by learning assertive responses, since assertive behaviors are incompatible with feelings of anxiety.

The terms "assertive training" or "assertion training" describe an approach like social skills training for helping persons to acquire or reestablish skills for expressing positive and negative feelings clearly. Social skills training is a more generic term that includes interpersonal goals that go beyond self-assertion. In the late 1960s Lazarus introduced the term "behavioral rehearsal" to describe a combination of modeling and roleplaying aimed at increasing patients' assertive behavior. Wolpe and Lazarus pointed out that individuals who could benefit from assertion training may have never learned how to show their anger and annoyance or may have been punished or ignored for expressing such feelings. Moreover, they argued that unassertive persons have become "conditioned" to responding to interpersonal situations with anxiety and passivity rather than clearly and openly expressing their feelings to others.

Salter, Wolpe, Lazarus, and other early pioneers in behavior therapy developed the basic procedures for teaching assertive behavior that enable patients to act in their own best interests, to stand up for themselves without undue anxiety, and to exercise their rights without denying the rights of others. Their important contributions were using learning theory and documenting that a practical clinically relevant technique could be used effectively by practitioners.

During the 1960s, applications of Skinner's research in operant conditioning led to an expansion of learning-based treatments for patients with deficient emotional and social communication skills. The focus of the remedial therapy shifted from individuals to groups and even to entire treatment units like wards in psychiatric hospitals, target populations expanded beyond mildly disturbed neurotic patients with anxiety and mood disorders to retarded persons, juvenile delinquents, and chronic psychotic inpatients and outpatients. In addition to self-assertion and standing up for one's rights, a broad spectrum of instrumental and affiliative skills was operationally defined and targeted for modification. Communication skills—rational and coherent speech, affection and tenderness, sadness and grief, heterosocial interactions, anger and empathy—were taught to patients in hospitals, clinics, and private offices.

Bandura's research in social learning led to the incorporation of modeling procedures into social skills training. Bandura and other behavioral scientists demonstrated that a range of emotions, from rage and aggression to tenderness and love, can be learned by observing and imitating a role model. Researchers of social learning described how the content of speech, arm and hand gestures, facial expressions, vocal tone and pace, and bodily movements combined to communicate feelings, and how each of these components was learned through observing appropriate models. For example, it was shown that persons judged high in assertiveness tended to speak longer in responses to questions, talk louder, request more information from others, and pause for shorter periods than did those who were judged to be unassertive.

In the 1970s a number of clinical researchers independently developed and validated methods for more systematically teaching people how to express their feelings and converse in social interactions. These teaching techniques were based upon principles of learning and incorporated the basic steps of modeling, behavioral rehearsal, positive social feedback, repeated rehearsal, homework, and generalization training in well-delineated therapy manuals. Different names were given to these structured teaching methods, including *social skills training, structured learning therapy,* and *personal effectiveness training*.

This decade of research witnessed a plethora of studies examining the utility of social skills training with a wide variety of clinical populations. The main results of these investigations were positive, showing that social skills training procedures were effective in teaching new skills and that these new skills often generalized to new situations for which the patient had not received training. However, not all behaviors were found to be equally generalizable to novel situations. Simple behaviors, such as eye contact, were found to generalize more readily than were complex behaviors, such as requesting changes in others' behavior. Difficulties in promoting generalization presented a dilemma for psychiatric patients, since they needed to use complex behaviors to obtain necessary resources and generate social support from others in a variety of community-based situations.

As research on the applications of social skills training mounted, it became increasingly clear that social skills were behaviors that could be taught to psychiatric patients with generalization and durability only by attending to patients' perceptual and cognitive skills. By the end of the 1970s a new model of social skills training had emerged that incorporated techniques to teach perceptual or receiving skills, cognitive or processing skills, and behavioral or sending skills. More refined research with psychiatric patients began to examine the efficacy of social skills training on diagnostically homogeneous groups of patients; in addition the effect of such training was examined on clinically standardized instruments of illness severity and social adjustment. In recent years, these more sophisticated methods of research and training of social skills have resulted in longer-lasting and broader improvements in patients' social skills and also in conferring protection against relapse.

ASSUMPTIONS OF SOCIAL
SKILLS TRAINING

A basic assumption of social skills training, supported by research evidence, is that the acquisition of the behavioral concomitant of an emotion is *followed* by the subjective experience of that emotion. For example, after several sessions of practicing the verbal, postural, gestural, vocal, and facial expressions that communicate interest and concern for another person, a patient who was initially socially withdrawn and anhedonic began to experience the gradual return of warmth, pleasure, and internal comfort in that relationship. Furthermore, focusing on the teachable and demonstrable signs of affective expression is a more efficient means of bringing about emotional change than is concentrating directly on the internal feeling states.

The subjective and physiological experiences of joy, pleasure, anger, assertiveness, tenderness, and affection develop following active practice and rehearsal of the behaviors that convey these feelings and by the positive feedback that clear and direct communications engender in significant others. Social skills trainers assume that changes in self-esteem and self-confidence, positive experiences, and subjective comfort will follow, rather than precede, changes in overt behavior. With this assumption, the main goal of social skills training is first to help the patient change his or her behavior in visible and audible ways. As these skills develop and improve, patients experience positive reactions in others with whom they interact and begin to feel better about themselves and their ability to achieve their interpersonal goals. Self-reinforcement and favorable reactions from others strengthen these skills, ensuring that they will remain in the patient's behavioral repertoire after training has ceased.

Another major assumption of social skills training with psychiatric patients concerns the relative availability and "richness" of social reinforcement in the environment where the patient resides. Bear in mind that deficits in skills are thought to be caused by either the lack of appropriate role models while growing up or the loss of skills due to the disruptive effects of the illness itself. Thus, while patients in any environment can be taught social skills, these skills will be retained and will generalize to novel situations only if the patients' social environment consistently reinforces the use of these skills. A minimum of such naturally occurring social reinforcement is essential to maintaining gains in social skills. The absence of rewarding social encounters will discourage patients from using their skills, leading to the disuse and withering away of newly acquired behaviors.

Social skills training cannot be clinically effective when provided in an environment devoid of interpersonal and material reinforcers. Thus, a schizophrenic patient who lives on Social Security Disability income, as an isolate in a subsidized apartment in a low-rent housing project, who has no relatives or friends, and who does not attend a day treatment program is unlikely to experience any long-term benefits from social skills training unless his or her environment is modified to make it more potentially rewarding. Similarly, a "back ward" psychiatric patient will be helped by social skills training only if rewarding interactions with other patients and with staff members are sufficiently available.

For social skills training to have any sustained impact on patient's functioning, steps must be undertaken to improve the availability of social reinforcement in the natural environment such as by counseling relevant family, friends, or other caregivers to respond positively and consistently to the patient's appropriate social behavior. Another useful strategy is to help the patient identify specific situations with greater potential for meaningful and rewarding interactions, such as recreation groups, day treatment centers, "drop-in" social clubs, or public activities that can give patients more control over their social environment.

HOW TO USE THIS GUIDEBOOK

This guidebook has been prepared so that people in the mental health, counseling, and rehabilitation fields can learn the specifics of social skills training and apply the procedures in the settings where they work, including hospitals, clinics, day treatment centers, private offices, community mental health centers, residential communities, and sheltered workshops. The guidebook has four sections:

1. *The assessment of social skills*, which covers methods for determining the assets and deficits of patients' social and independent living skills that lead to a prescription for skills training and clinical goals.
2. *The social skills training sequence*, including how to motivate and engage patients in goal setting, behavioral rehearsal, modeling, coaching, and homework assignments for improving "receiving," "processing," and "sending" skills.
3. *Teaching friendship and dating skills*, in which a structured module is described for helping a wide range of patients improve their ability to make friends and relate to members of the opposite sex.
4. *Dealing with special problems*, such as resistance to roleplaying and

teaching basic skills to thought disordered and low-functioning psychotic patients.

Detailed and graphic transcripts of therapist and patient interaction from real training sessions are provided throughout the guidebook so that the reader can grasp the underlying principles and specific techniques of social skills training. The guidebook should enable readers with experience as therapists and counselors to understand and apply the methods creatively within the context of their own programs and clinical styles. In fact, the techniques outlined for group leaders, counselors, or therapists will be enhanced by adapting them to fit the specific needs of the psychiatric population under treatment. Social skills training can be readily added to the existing repertoire of any practitioner's therapeutic skills. The methods are practical and pragmatic and do not require a commitment to a philosophy or theory of treatment and human behavior.

This guidebook provides clinical methods for professionals in the helping fields to assist psychiatric patients in developing more skillful ways of expressing feelings, getting ends met and making social contacts. Appropriate patients for skills training include psychiatric in-patients; chronically ill patients attending day hospitals, community support programs, or vocational rehabilitation programs; and those with mood, psychosomatic, or anxiety disorders seeking help privately or at community mental health centers. The methods described here can be employed in the context of individual, family, and group psychotherapy.

Social skills training is presently being carried out by psychiatric technicians, occupational therapists, psychiatric social workers, nurses, vocational counselors, rehabilitation therapists, psychologists, and psychiatrists. The procedures can be learned by virtually anyone in the mental health, educational, and rehabilitation fields. A careful reading of this guidebook will provide a comprehensive introduction to social skills training. While this guide will provide substantial information in the practical use of this type of therapy, successful application of the methods requires much clinical practice and experience. For this reason individuals beginning to use social skills training should have access to a qualified consultant who has knowledge and experience with the methods of social skills training and behavior therapy, and who can be called upon to provide training and supervision until competence is achieved. A demonstration video and an inservice training guide are available for instructional purposes from the first author.

Learning and conducting social skills training with psychiatric patients can be a very rewarding, enriching experience. We invite you to participate in the practice exercises in the subsequent chapters as they will provide experiential learning and a chance to form your own implementation plan for social skills training in your practice.

PRACTICE EXERCISES

1. Pinpointing the patient's assets and coping abilities, no matter how symptomatic, regressed, and low functioning he or she is, is a prerequisite for conducting goals in social skills training. From among your current clinical caseload or past clinical experience, select a patient with a major mental disorder. Then list the residual or continuing capabilities of this patient in such social and life spheres as family ties, peer relations, relationships with paraprofessionals, self-care skills, work, recreational activities, and emotional expression.

2. The stress-vulnerability-coping skills model of mental illness emphasizes the important role of stress in precipitating or worsening the symptoms of the illness. Furthermore, patients with good coping skills and social support are more successful at minimizing the untoward effects of stress on their psychobiological vulnerability. From your current or past caseload, choose two patients who have recently had symptom relapses. Make a list of the different types of stressors your patients had been exposed to prior to their relapses, including life events, a negatively charged social climate, overstimulation, lack of structure and understimulation, overly demanding expectations for behavior change, or inadequate material resources. For each stressor you identify, evaluate whether improved social skills and/or social support would have enabled the patient to cope more effectively with the stress. You will see that most potent stressors that impinge on psychiatric patients can be reduced by enhancing social skills and support.

3. Social skills training builds coping skills for patients to use in their interpersonal relations so they may better obtain their material and emotional needs. The focus of training is on the *coping skills*, while the desired outcomes of the patients' use of these skills can be said to reflect their *social competence*. Pick a patient for illustrative purposes and describe a coping or social skill that could help that person achieve some personal need or goal. Then describe how that goal, if achieved, would reflect a higher level of social competence for the person. If you carry out this exercise, you will readily see how multiplying a person's coping skills across many domains of life leads to cumulatively greater social competence and personal independence.

SUMMARY

Humans are social creatures who need to interact with others to meet their emotional, social, and biological needs. One of the most important reasons that psychiatric patients have so much difficulty obtaining their needs and coping with everyday life is their inability to express themselves effectively to others. Even when the most recognizable symptoms of mental illness are controlled by medication, patients' ability to communicate effectively remains impaired. In short most people with a major mental disorder have poor social skills, and social skills are the ingredients of effective communications.

Social interactions include three stages: receiving skills, that allow us to "size up" the situation and formulate an appropriate response; processing skills, that guide us in choosing the style and content of a good response; and sending skills, that are used in the actual delivery of the response. Social problem solving can be done with skills enabling individuals to search for, select, and implement the best way of dealing with interpersonal situations.

The style of communication is extremely important in determining personal effectiveness. The "how" of communication is made up of paralinguistic skills, such as voice volume (loudness), fluency and pacing of speech, intonation, and how quickly we respond when the other person stops talking; and nonverbal skills, including facial expression, hand gestures, body posture, eye contact and how near or far away we are from the other person when we are communicating with them.

Helping patients improve their social skills is vital. Research of the past twenty years points to the importance of the stress-vulnerability-coping skills model of mental illness, which holds that certain people are biologically vulnerable to psychiatric illness, that stressors in life can make it much more likely that the person will develop symptoms, and that medication, coping skills, and social support can buffer the noxious effects of stress and vulnerability. The major component of coping skills is social skills; therefore, proficiency in social skills protects against the symptoms and disabilities of mental disorders.

This guidebook describes an approach to training a wide spectrum of psychiatric patients in these skills. Social skills training is highly structured, fast moving, and rewarding to patients and therapists alike. The skills are taught in much the same way as other skills. Basic principles of human learning are applied with precision in this approach in the interest of efficiency and effectiveness. Modeling and imitation, sometimes called observational learning; setting positive expectations; positive reinforcement; and coaching; and transfer of learned skills to patients' natural life environments are harnessed together to maximize skill development and utilization.

Chapter 2
Assessing Social Skills

What type of patients are suitable for social skills training? What kinds of behavioral problems and psychopathology interfere with a patient's accessibility to social skills training? Social skills training is a relatively nonspecific technique, providing generic strengthening and protection against the stress and vulnerability associated with all mental disorders; hence there are no particular diagnostic groups for whom social skills training is not indicated. However, the types of social deficits associated with various disorders and the specific skills deficits possessed by a particular patient will point the therapist in the direction of individualizing the goals for training.

The first assessment question that needs to be answered is: "How can patients be selected who will be appropriate for social skills training?" The best rule of thumb in identifying patients for social skills training is to determine their ability to follow instructions and to pay attention in a structured learning process; that will take from 15 minutes to 90 minutes, depending upon whether the training is offered in individual or group sessions.

There are several factors that can contribute to such poor attentional ability that even the prompting and highly structured nature of social skills training will not "reach" certain patients. One type of psychopathology is incoherence and other forms of severe thought disorder, such as that experienced in schizophrenia, that interfere with basic interpersonal communication. If the patient cannot understand the therapist or be understood by the therapist, the basic form of social skills training will not be effective. Similarly, short-term memory problems—as are found in patients with organic mental disorders like Alzheimer's disease—will make learning so tiresome that patients and therapists alike will soon burn out. The frequent intrusion of psychotic symptoms of schizophrenia or affective disorder—mania, delusions, hallucinations, agitation, pacing, hand-wringing—may also prevent patients from paying attention to the training steps and assimilating the skills being practiced. It should be noted, however, that the structure, prompting, and positive feedback offered in social skills training can displace psychotic symptoms in many patients, enabling them to learn interpersonal skills. It may be necessary to "experiment" by exposing a psychotic patient to social skills training, to see how readily learning takes place, before deciding that the symptoms are too intrusive for further training efforts.

In general, it is better to bring the thought disorder, memory impairment, or psychotic symptoms under some reasonable degree of control—as through the judicious use types and doses of psychotropic medication—before proceeding with social skills training. For patients who are refractory to psychoactive mediation, an intensive form of social skills training, termed "attention-focusing skills" training, may be helpful. This technique is described briefly in Chapter 5 of this guidebook, but it is extremely costly to implement in terms of staff time and effort.

Another factor that can interfere with the requisite attention and instruction following of social skills training is the sedative side effects of many psychotropic drugs. The doses of antidepressants, antipsychotics, anxiolytics, and hypnotics can usually be titrated downward to reduce or eliminate sedation while still retaining therapeutic and prophylactic effectiveness. Thus, the skills trainer who becomes aware of possible medication side effects interfering with a patient's concentration and task orientation in the training session should be prepared to communicate with the prescribing physician and to educate the patient about the need for dosage regulation.

Some patients with schizophrenic and personality disorders will simply refuse to participate in social skills training or in any form of therapy for that matter. The so-called "young-adult chronic mental patient" refuses treatment but permits himself or herself to be "rescued" from calamitous situations. Patients without insight into their illness may view social skills training as tantamount to acknowledging that they are mentally ill. In such cases of negativism, it is best to proceed from the point of the view of the patient, that is, to discover what personal goals the patient has and to try to persuade the patient that these goals might be achieved or approximated through participation in social skills training.

Mark, a young man with schizophrenia, refuses to take antipsychotic medication or come to see a psychiatrist. However, he wants to continue living at home with his parents and have access to the family car. When it was suggested that these goals might be attained through his practicing ways of being more personally effective with his parents, he agreed to attend a social skills training session "just to see what goes on."

The following criteria may be used in determining whether a patient can comprehend and attend to the elements of social skills training. Can he or she

- Respond appropriately when asked his name, date of birth, and the current date?
- Use and understand simple sentences?
- Listen to another person for at least three to five minutes without interruption?
- Follow simple, three-step instructions such as "stand up, walk over to the person sitting by the table, and say 'hello'?"
- Interact in a small-group setting without talking to self, pacing, provoking others, yelling, or exhibiting other acting-out behaviors?
- Express a desire to improve the expressing of personal feelings such as anger, fear, happiness, and frustration and describe feelings in a given situation, for example, "I was upset when I lost my wallet"?

The therapist should consult with other senior staff in reviewing cases in which it is unclear if a patient meets these guidelines. Patients should receive the benefit of the doubt and participate in social skills training even if they only minimally meet these guidelines.

A Practical Approach to Assessment

Assessment of the social skills and social deficits of individuals undergoing social skills training is tightly interwoven with the training process. As the trainer or therapist observes the patient practicing verbal and nonverbal expressiveness in the *behavioral rehearsals* or roleplays, opportunities abound for detecting the patient's strengths and weaknesses in coping with the situation being rehearsed. Identifying the behavioral assets and deficiencies in the patient's performances, as he or she progresses through a sequence or series of skills training scenes and sessions, is one of the most important ways of conducting an assessment of social skills. The way in which assessment questions lead to answers that serve as the "fuel" for the training enterprise is depicted in the flow chart of Figure 2-1. Training techniques are applied with patients as directed by the assessment findings. Assessment is key in pointing to the needs to remediate the deficiencies and build on the assets demonstrated by the patient's skills in "receiving," "processing," and "sending" communications.

It is also desirable, however, to carry out a preliminary assessment of social skills and social deficits of patients prior to their actually rehearsing situations in the skills training session. Initial goals must be set, and scenes for roleplaying need to be articulated, even without the benefit of having observed the patient "in action." To accomplish the task of the

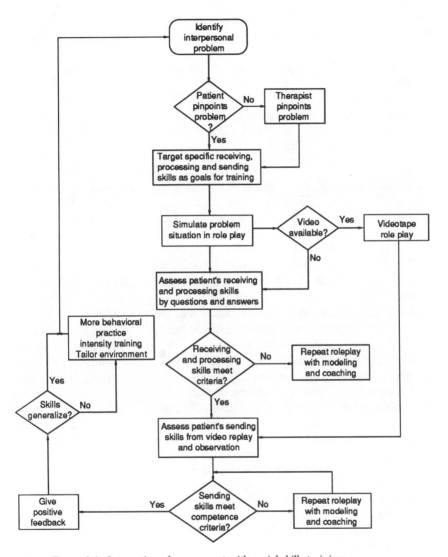

Figure 2-1. Integration of assessment with social skills training

initial assessment of social skills, the clinician must bring together all relevant sources of information. These include

- Psychiatric and social histories provided by the patient and other informants

- Previous medical and social service records
- Descriptions by the patient of the domains of functioning where interpersonal skills have been lacking
- Reports of the patient's social performance by other caregivers and relatives
- Observations of the patient's social interaction, communications, and relationships by clinical staff
- Rating forms and scales that can be completed by the patient or by others, including clinical staff

Thus, the social skills trainer has two major sources of information that can be funneled into the assessment of social skills and thence into the formulation and specification of interpersonal goals and situations that can be used in the training process per se. One source is the *behavioral rehearsal* that actually comprises part of the training steps; the other is the full spectrum of reports, biographical data, evaluations, and observations made about the patient, or by the patient, outside of the training setting.

Information from collaborating staff members, relatives, and significant others regarding the patient's social behaviors is especially important when the patient, because of the intrusion of symptoms, cognitive deficits, or lack of insight, cannot participate as a reliable informant during behavioral interviewing. For inpatients, the nursing staff is best positioned to observe the patient in naturalistic settings and give concrete descriptions of strengths and weaknesses, deficits of appropriate social skills, and excesses of maladaptive social behavior. Some examples of problems identified by nursing staff of patients with chronic and severe psychiatric disorders include

- Speaking only when spoken to
- Speaking in a monotone
- Making infrequent eye contact
- Begging, nagging, and pestering
- Making unreasonable demands
- Expressing disapproval through disruptive actions, such as yelling, swearing, making threatening gestures, and hitting
- Interrupting others impolitely
- Rambling on with delusional and irrelevant statements
- Failing to express needs or feelings on a regular basis to staff or peers
- Making inappropriate sexual advances, such as touching others in private areas, exposing self, or talking about sexual topics in a way that is embarrassing to others

- Crying often
- Making highly unrealistic statements about abilities and plans
- Constantly complaining
- Exhibiting great difficulty in initiating and maintaining simple day-to-day conversations
- Exhibiting any other behaviors that are considered socially unacceptable by the majority of "normal" adults or that are self-defeating and inhibit the patient from functioning like other "normal" adults in routine social interactions

In some skills training settings, it may not be feasible for the trainer to have had access to the full catalog of background information before having to plunge into goal setting and training itself. Meeting a new patient for the first time "cold," without even a referral note, need not be a cause for panic by the therapist. As is depicted in Table 2-1, the social skills therapist or trainer can elicit or formulate training goals with minimal assessment information if an inventory is taken of the patient's current capabilities in managing interpersonal transactions in affiliative and instrumental roles. Every patient, no matter how regressed or withdrawn, has opportunities for interpersonal contacts, and the adroit clinician can survey these and seize one or more as the focal point for a "dry run" behavioral rehearsal.

One format for social skills training that requires quick-witted clinical responsiveness and inquiries to assess skills and deficits and to establish training goals comes from drop-in or crisis intervention work with individuals, families, or groups. An example of social skills assessment and training in such brief therapy is the "Successful Living" group, which has been applied in community mental health centers and aftercare clinics at psychiatric hospitals. The following description of this open-ended social skills training group highlights the way goals can be set through clinical assessment.

A Successful Living group has been in operation for six years at the Brentwood (Psychiatric) Division of the West Los Angeles VA Medical Center. Its 1¹/₂-hour weekly sessions are open-ended in that attendance is encouraged beyond the first meeting, but is not mandatory. The group is advertised for drop-in or crisis intervention purposes, and the expectations are that each patient can accomplish something tangible—however modest—in even one session.

The group sessions open with a three-minute orientation in which the leader or therapist describes the aims, format, and rationale of the social skills training approach to solving interpersonal problems. An educa-

Table 2-1. Instrumental and Affiliative Roles That Serve as Domains for Eliciting or Setting Interpersonal Goals After Conducting a Social Skills Assessment

Role Domain	Assessed Deficit	Articulated Interpersonal Goal
Affiliative		
Family	Gets aggressive or withdraws sullenly when parent exhibits intrusiveness or emotional overinvolvement	To express need for privacy and autonomy in assertive manner
	Lack of transportation and unable to request assistance from parents	To tell parents how helpful it would be to borrow the family car
	Lack of cohesion in family ties and little or no positive exchanges	To express appreciation to mother for fine meals
Friends	No friends, socially isolated	To call an old friend on the phone and say hello
	Living in new residence, feels lonely and knows no one	To introduce self to three new people living in same place
	Wishes to have a girlfriend or boyfriend but has limited dating experience	To invite a female neighbor for coffee
Instrumental		
Job finding	Does not know how to elicit job leads	To ask three friends and three relatives if they know of any job openings
	Anxious using the telephone	To call a firm advertising a job and ask for information
	Reluctant to expose psychiatric history in job interview	To roleplay a job interview with counselor explaining lapses in employment as "personal development" periods
Recreation and leisure	Lacks interest and motivation to pursue recreational activities	To invite a friend to attend a movie or go bowling

tional, realistic, and upbeat tone for the sessions is established at the outset, and cohesion is promoted by having group members discuss problem solving with each other's problems, assisting each other in the training steps, and occasionally carrying out homework assignments as "buddies."

Patients are actively assisted in formulating goals in both affiliative and instrumental roles. New and returning patients alike are encouraged to select specific, current interpersonal problems to work on—in such domains as asserting one's needs with a health care provider, presenting oneself for a counseling session with a vocational rehabilitation counselor, obtaining payment on a debt from a roommate, going through a job interview, obtaining information on eligibility for Social Security benefits, and initiating conversations with strangers.

Some problems that do not necessarily seem interpersonal in context can usually be recast as such; for example, a patient who complains about a lack of adequate housing can be encouraged to roleplay a scene with a social worker whose responsibilities include assistance with residential placements. A patient who complains of trouble concentrating on his college coursework can be encouraged to practice asking for help from a tutor, teacher, or college counselor.

Translating problems and goals into interpersonal terms is a crucial and challenging assessment step for patient and therapist alike. While some patients want to identify areas requiring improvement in their social contacts and relations, others complain of a vague assortment of life burdens and may have little or no idea of how to proceed in articulating their problems in specific interpersonal themes and priorities. Such patients require guidance and direction from the therapist, who can help identify social interaction problems and goals by obtaining background information from the referring agent, relatives, and caregivers or by systematically interviewing the patient about his or her life. For example, a 53-year-old man with alcoholic hallucinosis, mystified by his diagnosis, was helped to formulate the goal of asking his doctor about his diagnosis and prognosis. A 29-year-old woman with a diagnosis of schizophrenia, who complained about not having enough money to meet her basic needs, agreed to a goal of saying no to unreasonable requests by friends and relatives for loans.

INSTRUMENTAL AND AFFILIATIVE SKILLS

Social skills can be functionally separated into those that have value in instrumental roles and situations and those that are helpful in mediating affiliative relationships. Instrumental skills enable a person to attain independence and material benefits, such as money, residence, goods, and services. Affiliative skills make it possible for an individual to make friends, enjoy intimacy, obtain emotional support, exhibit warmth, and engage in reciprocity with friends and relatives.

For practical purposes, drawing distinctions between interpersonal skills relevant for instrumental and affiliative roles is not important for the clinician intending to conduct social skills training. However, it is helpful for the clinician to have a clear understanding of the nature of these domains of role functioning so that assessment can readily be performed and relevant interpersonal goals constructed. The clinician should strive toward having a checklist, at the ready in his or her mind's eye, of a spectrum of interpersonal goals that can remediate deficits or excesses of social behavior in affiliative and/or instrumental areas of functioning.

Remember that social skills are the ability to give and obtain information and to express and exchange attitudes, opinions, and feelings in a wide variety of situations. The patient's short- and long-term goals, inherent in the situations, determine whether affiliative or instrumental needs are being dealt with and met. In instrumental roles and situations, social interaction serves to gain tangible ends that are required for physical, material, and financial well-being. Instrumental relationships thus have as their function the performance of tasks and the achievement of productive goals; work and service relationships primarily subserve instrumental role needs. Such interpersonal relationships as boss-employee, conductor-musician, teacher-student, clerk-customer, apartment manager–renter, agent-client, and doctor-patient serve instrumental goals. Even within families, aspects of the relationship between spouses or between parents and offspring serve instrumental role purposes—for example, when spouses discuss the division of labor in carrying out household tasks. The nature and quality of any interpersonal relationship affect and are affected by the attainment of instrumental goals and completion of tasks. In addition, the goals and tasks themselves govern instrumental interactions.

Examples of instrumental situations are

- Purchasing an item in a store
- Asking for directions for a bus trip
- Requesting a job promotion or salary raise
- Complaining about side effects from a drug and asking for relief from one's physician
- Giving information about work experiences at a job interview
- Inquiring about an apartment for rent
- Talking with a social worker about Social Security benefits

Instrumental situations require interpersonal communication of varying degrees of complexity, intimacy, duration, and frequency. Some situations can be managed with a single, brief question, while others may require repeated interactions, some with great intensity of expression, over a long period of time.

Carol, in her mid-20s, first developed schizophrenic symptoms in her late teens and has required three hospitalizations for relapses of her delusions and hallucinations. Once again, her psychotic symptoms are in remission but she has been apathetic, indolent, and socially withdrawn. She lives with her parents, who are very solicitous and caring, but there is tension in the home. They are getting impatient with her reclusiveness and her remaining in bed for much of the day. She complains that her parents treat her like a child, alternating between controlling everything she does and pressuring her to "get out and do things."

Carol and her parents are enrolled in a family education program where they are learning constructive ways of communicating with one another. From those sessions, it was decided that Carol would benefit from joining a social skills training group to assist her in setting and achieving personal goals. Carol has expressed a desire to get a job, but she has lost several previous jobs because of an inability to ask for instructions and an intolerance of any criticism from her employers. She gets easily frustrated and has acquired a defeatist attitude about work. Avoidance of the stress and depression that have been associated with jobs is one reason why Carol has been secluding herself at home.

Moreover, her awkwardness and inexperience in dealing with authority figures also extends to people who work in agencies, public transportation, shops, banks, and other places of business. She has not learned to fend for herself in the community and has never even learned to take advantage of the city bus system. When faced with learning to deal with the wider community, Carol becomes anxious and resistive.

While Carol and her parents need to reduce family stress by learning affiliative communication skills, both family problems and Carol's longer-term needs for autonomy will benefit when she learns to use instrumental skills outside the home.

The second sphere that encompasses human interaction is the affiliative or social-emotional one. In social-emotional situations, individuals don't need to acquire information or tangible items that will improve their physical or economic well-being, but rather are aiming to meet their affiliative needs through making acquaintances, conversing with friends and relatives, communicating emotions and experiences with intimates, and interacting with members of their immediate household. A social-emotional relationship is formed solely for the purpose of fulfilling itself—such as in love, marriage, or friendship. The transactions in such relationships are information, opinions, and feelings that are not necessarily aimed at accomplishing some tangible goal. Social-emotional interactions deal with expressions of love, hate, sympathy, ambivalence, warmth, alienation, concern, sadness, happiness, and wishes. The major targets or goals of social-emotional situations are to acquire, make more intimate, and maintain friendships and family relationships.

Examples of social-emotional situations are

- asking one's spouse how he or she feels
- disciplining one's child
- greeting a friend with a hug and a smile
- complaining to one's spouse about feeling tired or ill
- going to a show with a friend
- asking one's neighbor whom he or she will vote for
- exchanging comments with an acquaintance about an illness, the weather, or sports

Obviously some interpersonal interactions serve both instrumental and social-emotional functions, such as when a father praises his child for carrying out a chore or errand. It is not the interpersonal "other" that defines the nature of the interaction; rather, it is the primary function of the specific interaction for the individuals concerned. In some situations, one person is obtaining gratification of instrumental needs while the other person is obtaining social-emotional satisfaction. This can occur when a person agrees to drive a neighbor to the hospital in an emergency and receives thanks and gratitude in return. The driver has succeeded in strengthening the friendship ties with his or her neighbor (social-emotional needs) and the neighbor has obtained needed medical care (instrumental needs). The family, in previous generations and in more traditional societies, satisfied both instrumental and social-emotional needs. In recent years, however, the family has satisfied fewer instrumental needs, since geographical and social mobility as well as other factors have preempted the work and economic functions of the family.

The following vignettes describe real patients who have participated in social skills training. For each patient described, note the assets and deficits delineated in social skills as well as the specific interpersonal goals and roleplay scenes which were formulated for the training process.

Case Vignette	Social Skills Assets and Deficits	Interpersonal Goals
Carol, described earlier, is experiencing negative symptoms of schizophrenia and verbalizes a desire to overcome her apathy and social anxiety. She would like to find employment, but is concerned about another job failure.	Speaks clearly with good intonation but has expressionless face and is stiff and tremulous. She tends to avoid or flee any socially stressful encounter.	Say "hello" and "thank you" to clinic secretary and clerks at stores; ask for information about volunteering at local Senior Citizen's Center on the telephone.

Ted, a 27-year-old electronics assembler with a borderline personality disorder, has great difficulty sustaining friendships with men and women. He is easily irritated and tends to misinterpret others' actions as trying to exploit or hurt him. He has been arrested twice for fighting in bars.

Has excellent nonverbal skills—very expressive in voice and face. Far too easily angered because of poor "receiving" or social perception skills. Lacks conflict resolution and negotiation skills.

Ask co-workers to describe and elaborate their opinions and ideas before jumping to conclusions. Give supervisor a compliment.

Karen, a 39-year-old mother of two young boys, has had recurrent major depressions superimposed on a chronic dysthymic disorder. She is at times desperate and suicidal as she feels hopeless about the future. Antidepressant medication has improved her mood, but she remains awkward, shy, and anxious with others outside of her home. She has trouble going to the store and has been out of contact with her friends for many months.

Wants to improve social skills to be a better mother and wife, able to intervene decisively with children; speaks in monotone and has flat facial expression. Poor at generating options for solving problems.

Request husband to compliment her cooking and child management efforts at least three times a week; phone her best friend and say that she is feeling better.

Alan was first diagnosed as having schizophrenia at the age of 15 when his teachers noted that he remained totally aloof from his classmates, rocked in his chair, and talked to himself. He

Is sensitive to social stimuli, and affected by others. Averts eye contact, mumbles, monotone voice, poverty of speech.

Respond to simple questions with one- or two-sentence answers, without rocking, and loudly enough to be heard 3 feet away.

responded to questions in a monotone and with monosyllabic answers. When relatives or nursing staff attempted to engage him in conversation, his rocking increased in speed, he bit into his fingers, and he destroyed his clothing and nearby furniture. He moved from one psychiatric hospital to another, but after being involved in a social learning token economy program, showed substantial improvement in his sociability. Now he lives in a board-and-care home and visits his family on weekends. He'd like to move back home full time.

Tell his family how much he enjoys his weekend visits.

Carl drifted in an apathetic life-style for a year after his discharge for a florid schizophrenic episode with auditory hallucinations and incoherence. He spent his days lying on the sofa at home watching TV. If his sister did not wake him up and drive him to the day treatment center he did not attend. Shortly after meeting a girlfriend who was well organized and supportive, Carl found a part-time job, took an interest in his appear-

Initiates contacts with friends; able to develop intimate heterosexual relationship; able to obtain a job and an apartment.

Lacks knowledge about his illness and need for maintenance antipsychotic drugs; not able to obtain information from health care providers or negotiate medication issues with doctor.

Exchange self-disclosures in equitable and balanced way with roommate.

Describe side effects from neuroleptic drugs specifically to doctor.

Negotiate medication dosage, adjustment with doctor.

ance, purchased new clothes, and began working out with weights. He moved out of his family home and found a roommate. For the first time in almost two years he seemed "alive," energetic, and goal directed. This lasted about two months. In quick succession, he got the "flu," lost his job, broke up with his girlfriend, and grieved the accidental death of a friend. While agreeing to increase his dose of neuroleptic medication, Carl surreptitiously stopped taking it. Within a few weeks he became psychotic and was rehospitalized.

Joe was 30-years-old and a successful dentist; however, he lacked communication skills with his wife and assertive skills with his dental partner, which allowed grievances to build up without remedy. He ultimately had a major depression and recovered slowly with cognitive behavior therapy and antidepressant medication.

Engages in small talk well with patients and acquaintances; able to reward and discipline his children.

Is unable to exchange intimate positive or negative feelings with spouse; withdraws from all conflict or discussion with partner over disagreements.

To acknowledge pleasing behavior of wife; to make positive requests for more frequent sex and companionship with wife; to do verbal problem solving with dental partner.

GUIDELINES FOR SETTING INTERPERSONAL GOALS IN SOCIAL SKILLS TRAINING

Some situations involving person-to-person communication make better goals for social skills training than others. Using selection criteria in goal setting is particularly important when starting social skills training and when working with inept and inexperienced patients. Several criteria can be used to determine which of several possible scenes should be chosen. Goals and situations should be formulated that are

1. *Attainable*; for example, making small talk with an attractive person *before* asking for a date, giving a compliment *before* expressing disagreement, asking boss for positive feedback on job performance *before* asking for a raise.

2. *Positive and constructive behaviors*; for example, asking for help in improving one's job performance as opposed to talking back to a boss, requesting a desired change in the actions of a spouse instead of arguing or complaining about past unpleasantness.

3. *Specific*; that is, the goal must be described in concrete interpersonal terms: *what* emotion or need is to be communicated? with whom? where? and when? (e.g., "I would like to be able to approach strangers at the park or beach and exchange some greeting or comment about the weather or the immediate situations.")

4. *Functional behaviors*; that is, they should provide maximum payoff for the patient in the real world. For example, asking a friend to lunch as opposed to asking for a favor, expressing affection as opposed to criticism, requesting a job interview rather than talking with a staff member.

5. *Consistent with the patient's rights and responsibilities*; that is, the goal should conform to socially expected behavioral norms and not violate family or subcultural values. For example, the appropriate and expected use of eye contact with individuals considered in superior status differs between cultures—Anglo-American, Mexican, Asian. The anticipated response from the other person should likewise dovetail with norms and social rules.

6. *Chosen by the patient*; that is, whatever structuring and suggestions for goals come from the therapist, family, and other caregivers, the patient should be solicited to participate in the goal setting to the maximum degree feasible.

7. *High-frequency behaviors*; that is, those that frequently occur and can be practiced often. For example, initiating conversations as opposed to returning defective merchandise, asking a boss to repeat instructions

rather than asking for a raise, greeting a spouse warmly at the end of each day rather than waiting for a birthday or anniversary.

8. *Likely to occur in the near future or have occurred in the recent past*; in other words, it is best to select goals for training that are fresh and salient for the patient's current life situation.

Some examples of desirable and undesirable goals for social skills training are given in Table 2-2.

Allen, now 22-years-old, has responded minimally to antipsychotic medication. He remains extremely withdrawn, exhibits peculiar mannerisms, and talks to his "voices." In previous social skills training, he has learned to tolerate conversational contacts with others, to make appropriate eye contact, and to speak in brief sentences. He no longer acts out destructively and has been able to live at home with his parents and younger sister. He attends a partial hospitalization program three days a week in addition to the weekly social skills training group.

Goals for the social skills training were set collaboratively by Allen, his

Table 2-2. Criteria and Examples of Desirable and Undesirable Behavioral Goals for Social Skills Training

Criteria	Desirable Goals	Undesirable Goals
Positive and constructive	Ask teacher for help Give a report in a conference fluently	Stop talking back to Reduce social anxiety and public speaking phobia
Functional	Describe past work history in job interview Invite friend for coffee Give affection to spouse	Speak up in group therapy Invite therapist for coffee Express feelings to therapist
High frequency	Give praise to child for school achievement Converse with co-workers at lunch break	Hug child on birthday Converse with co-workers at annual company picnic
Attainable	Talk for one minute with female sales clerk in store Ask husband to help with dishes	Ask a pretty girl out for a date Ask husband to babysit children
Specific	Initiate three conversations with strangers during week Make daily phone calls to elicit job leads	Be more sociable Search for job
Consistent with rights and responsibilities	Request that physician provide information about side effects and benefits of medication	Demand that doctor change prescription
Current in patient's life	Explain lapses in employment record in forthcoming job interview	Express anger at previous boss for being laid off job

family, and the staff of the partial hospitalization program. As a first step it was decided that Allen could learn how to offer to help with chores at home, and a specific one was chosen, namely, to offer to help in preparing the evening meal. This goal was *attainable*, as his family readily agreed to respond favorably to his offer to help with chores; it was *positive and constructive*; it represented a *functional* activity because it showed the family that Allen could be helpful and sociable, thereby reducing the tension that had built up by Allen's social isolation and almost incessant TV watching; it was *chosen*, at least in part, by Allen who preferred cooking to housecleaning; and it was in the domain of *high-frequency* behavior because chores could be done on a daily basis.

PRACTICE EXERCISE

Either on your own or with a colleague decide upon interpersonal goals and scenes that could be used in training social skills for the patients described in the paragraphs that follow. Be sure you have chosen, to the greatest extent possible, goals whose behaviors are specific, attainable, positive, functional, within the patient's normative rights and responsibilities, and occur at a high frequency.

Ann is a college sophomore having difficulty standing up for her opinions and ideas in class even when she is sure she is correct. In other situations, she doesn't have this problem.

Russ has a hard time asking favors of people. This is his third social skills training session. He failed to carry out an assignment to ask several people for matches. He wished to practice asking a neighbor to drive him to a garage to pick up his car.

Jim is a new student who has a difficult time expressing affection toward his wife.

Felicia's husband always decides what they will watch on TV, and Felicia would like to be able to watch some shows that she prefers.

LaVerne's former landlord has refused to return her cleaning deposit of $50.00 and claims that she has damaged things that were already damaged when she moved in. LaVerne would like to practice the scene with a female; her landlord is a male.

Robert is a relatively new patient who seems to be very shy and withdrawn. He rarely initiates conversations with staff or other patients.

Dorothy would like to be able to accept and give criticism more

(continued)

easily. She is rather adamant about roleplaying with only one particular patient in the social skills training group.

Jacob is a new student who has had trouble "selling himself" in job interviews. He is eager to work on his interaction.

Danny has difficulty expressing his anger reasonably. He is making good progress and would like to work on a scene involving his reaction to a waiter's spilling coffee on him.

Sue socializes poorly; she is unable to ask others to do things with her (e.g., going to the movies, shopping). This is her second social skills training session, but she is reluctant to do a scene.

GETTING SPECIFIC

The most challenging step in social skills training is assisting the patient in formulating the goals, situations, and specific interpersonal scenes that will be used for the training process. To the maximum extent feasible, patients should be encouraged to participate actively in selecting their goals and in designing the particular scene that will be rehearsed in the subsequent training session. Clinicians can be most helpful in facilitating the goal setting toward attainable and functional "targets" if they bring to the planning process information on the patient's past history and life adjustment, family reports, interview and medical record data, summaries of past treatment experiences, and observations on the patient's social behavior made by other treating professionals. Thus, if at all possible, the clinician should come to a training session armed with a grasp of the patient's interpersonal and expressive assets and deficits and then plan the patient's choice of goals and scenes in light of this knowledge. But the most powerful means of enlisting the patient's collaboration in identifying goals for social skills training comes from the kinds of questions that are asked at this point in the process.

By asking highly pointed and focused questions, you will be successful in bringing your patients from a preoccupation with their general problems, symptoms, disabilities, and dysphoria to a level of constructive specificity that will permit the development of goals and scenes for training. But what guidelines are to be used for the questions? Consider the stress-vulnerability-skills model presented in Chapter 1, because it will give direction to fruitful sources of questioning. Questioning can be pursued that elucidates the *stressors* experienced by patients, their current *coping efforts to deal with stress, efforts aimed at maintaining or improving social functioning* and their *quality of life and social support networks,* and interpersonal transactions that could *"displace" or reduce* their current severity of *symptoms.*

Coping With Stressors

Questions can be asked that help the patient to pinpoint stressors that are impinging on them and, if dealt with more effectively, could be decompressed or detoxified. There are two kinds of stressors that should be taken into account: (1) *time-limited life events* that have a definite beginning and end (e.g., loss of job or getting a new job; discharge from hospital or termination by therapist or doctor, or change in therapist or doctor; move to a new residence; episode of drinking alcohol or using street drugs that exacerbates symptoms; not receiving one's Social Security Disability check on time) and (2) *ambient tensions and conflicts* that arise from ongoing relationships at work, or with friends and family (e.g., overstimulating round of socializing, emotionally overarousing social or sexual intimacy, excessively high performance demands at work or home, repeated criticism from boss or family member, emotional overinvolvement with relative or friend). Thus, the following types of questions could be asked to help a patient articulate these sources of stress:

- What upsetting experience or event preceded your last relapse or led to your admission to the hospital?
- What kinds of changes have occurred in your life recently, such as moving your home, changes in contact with friends or relatives, changes in the professionals who are assisting you, changes in your schedule of activities?
- Do you feel tension or conflict in your home with your relatives? At work? At school? In your relationship with your therapist or in the hospital or clinic?
- Are any of your relationships too close for comfort?
- Is there anyone that expects more from you than you can realistically achieve or do?
- Have you been influenced by friends to use alcohol or drugs against your better judgment?

One of the most important sources of stress for psychiatric patients with severe and disabling disorders comes from the strain and tension within the family. Studies from several countries have documented a robust relationship between the emotional climate in the family home and the likelihood of relapse in patients with depression, schizophrenia, mania or anorexia nervosa. In trying to deal with baffling and unremitting mental disorders, family members often fail to obtain information and advice from mental health caregivers. Without education, relatives may not recognize the existence of a bona fide biomedical disorder in the patient, or they may attempt to compensate for the patient's disability by overinvolvement, excessive nurturance, and overprotectiveness. Excessive criticism and emotional overinvolvement are the main stress factors that lead to relapse in vulnerable patients.

When a patient who appears physically sound fails to function, it is perhaps understandable that relatives might grow frustrated and criticize the patient's failure to perform. In fact, relatives who are overinvolved or critical of their sick family member often express dissatisfaction with the patient's reluctance to converse, his or her apathy and social withdrawal, and his or her behavioral unpredictability. These behavioral targets for relatives' stressful relations can be viewed as social skills deficits in the patient.

Therefore, one way to reduce the adverse effects of family stress would be to develop goals for the disabled psychiatric patient to pursue in social skills training. Skills in the patient that could be trained for improving his or her adaptation within the family might include (1) developing social contacts outside the home, that is, peer relationships, involvement in social clubs, and vocational and prevocational skills; (2) learning to become more assertive with those relatives who are critical and overly involved, for example, asking for privacy, establishing one's own rights and responsibilities in the home, reinforcing relatives' positive comments, ignoring or escaping from relatives' critical comments or intrusiveness; and (3) teaching relatives and patients together to positively reinforce each other's desired behaviors and to rechannel criticism and overinvolvement toward constructive problem solving and mutual autonomy; for example, patient inviting relatives to attend an educational session with the doctor to learn more about the disorder.

Ted, to whom you've been introduced, has decided to seek counseling for his repeated difficulties with friends and co-workers. Getting arrested for disorderly conduct, after an altercation in a bar, was the final straw that motivated him to seek help; the judge agreed to place him on probation without a fine or jail sentence if he would obtain professional help. In his first evaluation session at the mental health center, he is interviewed by a psychiatric social worker who asks

Therapist: Ted, what are the kinds of things that happen in a bar that lead up to the fracases you've had?

Ted: Well, I drink more than I should. I'm always more touchy and grouchy when I'm loaded. I know I shouldn't drink so much, but my buddy can hold liquor better than I can, and I try to keep up with him.

Therapist: I see. Then what happens to start the arguments?

Ted: People will look at me and say something, and I feel like they're putting me down. I give 'em a mean look back and tell 'em to shove it.

One thing leads to another, and before I know it, punches are being thrown.

Therapist: Do you feel put down at other places, too? Where else do you have this kind of problem?

Ted: At work.

Therapist: Who gives you a hard time or hassles you? Who do you have a problem getting along with?

Ted: My supervisor, Mr. Houk. He's always coming around and poking his nose into my work. He usually doesn't say nothin', but I know he's thinking bad things about me. He just doesn't like me. He's too strict with everybody. For instance, he don't let nobody listen to music or anything while we're working.

Notice how the therapist solicited very specific information from Ted that provided clues about the kinds of stressors, as well as the deficits in social skills, that were likely to be incriminated in Ted's behavioral problems. Rather than spending time analyzing the "whys" of Ted's interpersonal problems, the therapist instead asked "what?" "where?" and "with whom?" types of questions. This brief interview productively yielded several possible goals and scenes for social skills training:

- Learning to be more accurate in decoding and reading the intent and feeling states of others—especially facial expressions.
- Saying "no" when invited to go drinking; suggesting alternate outlet for recreational activity with his buddy.
- Requesting a soft drink from the bartender.
- Expressing annoyance or irritation with words instead of with fists.
- Making efforts to improve the quality of the work relationship with Mr. Houk, as through the communication skills of "giving positive feedback" and "making a positive request."

Which of the possible goals and associated scenes a therapist might choose to use in social skills training with Ted will depend upon the criteria delineated in Table 2-2. Usually, a good place to begin training is with a situation that is not too demanding or too stressful and is therefore more likely to yield success. Success builds greater confidence for the patient to undertake more challenging interpersonal situations and relationships. Thus, it might be advisable to begin with improving his work relationship with Mr. Houk because it is less tinged by the additional arousing influence of alcohol and is more functional for Ted's meeting his needs for maintaining a job.

We will return to Ted in the next chapter and see how this assessment information is used in the training per se.

Building Upon Current Coping Skills

Another useful sector to probe with questions involves use of the coping skills that patients have to maintain their current life-style or to improve upon it. Questions such as the following can be used to target feasible points of departure for social skills training:

- What kinds of changes might you make in your life to bring yourself more satisfaction and sense of accomplishment? At work? With your family? With friends? With becoming more independent?
- How would you like your life to be different from the way it is now?
- Are there people you would like to become more friendly with? Do things with? Improve your relationship with?
- What situations in your everyday life do you avoid because of feeling inadequate, anxious, or lacking in confidence?

Almost everyone can benefit from efforts to enrich their quality of life, so these types of questions are fairly generic for all patients. After finding an area for which improvement (or consolidation and strengthening) is desired, then your task again requires asking "what?" "with whom?" "when?" "where?" and "what would happen then?" types of questions to get the necessary level of specificity for a scene to use in the ensuing rehearsals.

Let's try to highlight some areas and scenes for improving the quality of life and personal independence for Carol, who has already been introduced to you in the text.

Therapist: Carol, what sorts of changes would you like to see take place in your life?

Carol: There's so much wrong with me now, I can't think of just one or two things. I'm unhappy and uptight almost all of the time.

Therapist: You're feeling low, without energy, and anxious in part because your life has been rather empty lately. Let's see where you can begin to have some success in doing things; then, you'll gradually feel better about yourself.

Carol: I'd really like to move out of my folks' home and live in my own apartment.

Therapist: What would you need to have before you could take that step?

Carol: Money. A job, I guess.

Therapist: You're right! Independence costs money, and the way we can get enough money for an apartment is through working. But it's been a long time since you've held a job, and we don't want you to add more stress to yourself than you can handle right now. Can you think of something that might be like a regular job? You know, some activity that would give you the hang of working again but would be fairly low-key and easy to manage?

Carol: I spoke to the Vocational Rehab Counselor about going to the sheltered workshop, but I don't like the idea of working with people who are mentally retarded.

Therapist: Can you think of some other place where you can get some work experience, but without the stress of a real paying job?

Carol: I guess I could volunteer someplace for a few hours a day. Like at the General Hospital or Red Cross.

Therapist: Terrific idea, Carol. Let's see how we might help you achieve that first step toward independence here in social skills training.

Research conducted on a variety of psychiatric populations has led to conflicting results regarding the benefits afforded by social support networks in protecting patients against stress-induced relapse. One reason for the lack of consensus has been the failure by most investigators to measure the quality of the relationships and interactions that comprise a person's social support network. It should be obvious that the absolute numbers of social contacts, or even the degree to which relationships offer nurturance and assistance, are not as important as protective factors as are the nature, results, and outcomes of the interpersonal transactions. For example, family relations marked by emotional overinvolvement, where a parent or spouse offers excessive solicitude and concern for a mentally ill relative, can actually increase the risk of relapse—as well as reduce the opportunities for the ill person to develop his or her own independent capacities. Thus, if you have a patient who is experiencing too much social support, you might consider targeting assertiveness skills as a goal for social skills training. Your patient could request greater privacy from his or her relative, help from his or her relative in reaching goals that will serve as intermediate steps toward more independence, or less intrusiveness and protectiveness from relatives.

Goals That Displace Symptoms

Most of us have experienced how our social, recreational, and work activities displace tension, aches and pains, and minor symptoms of depression and anxiety. The fatigued and tense executive who returns home after a frustrating day at the office will feel a "pickup" of emotion if he or she spends the evening with friends watching football on TV or playing cards. A harried mother and housewife will find hidden resources of energy and enthusiasm if her husband takes her out to dinner and a show. Likewise with patients who have more persisting and intrusive symptoms—such as depression, anxiety, or hallucinations—engagement in activities that are keyed to their level of functioning and capabilities will often supplant symptoms and disabilities, albeit temporarily.

The kinds of questions that can offer leads to appropriate types of diversionary activities include

- What kinds of hobbies or recreational activities did you enjoy before you became ill?
- If you didn't suffer from depression (anxiety, hallucinations), what types of activities might you choose to participate in? Which people would you want to spend time with?
- What do you do to get temporary relief from your symptoms? Can you think of any times in the past week when you were free of symptoms, even for an hour?
- What kinds of activities and relationships do your symptoms prevent you from doing and seeing?

Finding an appropriate level of activity that will succeed in displacing or alleviating symptoms often takes some trial and experimentation. You can invite your patient to do this experimenting in a collaborative way with you, joining in the process of evaluating the benefits achieved from each effort to use some type of social skill. Here are some examples of the types of behavioral goals that can be used in social skills training to displace psychopathology in various types of disorders:

Agoraphobic woman . . .	makes a positive request of her husband to accompany her on a walk in the neighborhood and then, after her anxiety subsides, to return home alone to await her repeating the walk on her own.
Teenage girl suffering from hysterical dizziness . . .	assertively tells boyfriend that she does not wish to engage in sexual relations before marriage.
Depressed housewife recovering slowly from a suicide attempt . . .	asks her husband to attend a movie with her and go for an ice cream sundae afterwards, an activity they used to enjoy prior to her depression.
Drug abuser . . .	invites "straight" friends to engage in physical activities like sports when feeling a yen or craving for drugs.

Schizophrenic with bizarre posturing . . .	requests assistance from occupational therapist in learning a craft activity.
Socially isolated schizotypal patient . . .	phones a former friend and sets up a time to go shopping together.
Passive-aggressive person . . .	expressing annoyance directly and appropriately.
Schizoid personality . . .	initiates two-minute conversations with neighbors and relatives three times daily.

Allen experiences persistent and intrusive hallucinations that have been largely refractory to various types and doses of antipsychotic medication. His therapist enlists his involvement in setting a goal for social skills training.

Therapist: Allen, let's try to help you reduce the interference in your life that comes from the voices you hear, your hallucinations. If you get involved in some constructive activity that is within your ability to accomplish, you should be troubled less by the voices. The more you concentrate on the task or activity, the less you'll be bothered by the voices. OK?

Allen: But I don't feel like doing anything. I can't pay attention to even a TV program without those darn voices talking about me.

Therapist: Watching TV is kind of passive. Let's figure out an activity that will keep your attention and that you can succeed at. What sort of things did you enjoy doing or spend a lot of free time doing before you were 15-years-old?

Allen: I used to bake cookies and help in the kitchen. I liked it, but when I told my friend, he called me a sissy and made fun of me. So I stopped it.

Therapist: Nowadays, a lot of men are cooking as a hobby. That might be an activity that can put a lid on your voices. You're going home this weekend for a visit with your family, so why not practice in our social skills training session how to ask your mother to help out making something in the kitchen.

Allen: Won't the other people in the group make fun of that?

Therapist: I can assure you they won't. Let me tell you something: I cook and bake for a hobby, too. It takes my mind off my work and helps me relax.

As you can see from the flow chart in Figure 2-1, you must be prepared to assess the accuracy of the patient's social perception and flexibility in developing alternative responses to handle a problem situation. These domains are termed "receiving" and "processing" skills and are as important in achieving successful social outcomes as the verbal and nonverbal expressiveness of the patient.

PRACTICE EXERCISE

Select a patient from your caseload—current or past—who would be likely to benefit from social skills training. Go through this exercise on goal setting as a preliminary actually to employing the training steps you will learn about in the next chapter.

- Does the patient meet the criteria for a reasonable candidate for social skills training? Are there cognitive or symptom impairments that may interfere with learning?
- What sources of information can you use to inventory the patient's social skills assets and deficits?
- List the patient's instrumental and affiliative skills and the ways in which you might use social skills training to expand or strengthen these already existing skills.
- Select one initial goal that is highly specific to an interpersonal situation, identifying the "what?" "with whom?" "where?" and "when?" of the situational goal.
- What immediate goals would the patient be accomplishing if he or she used good skills in the situation? How would these short-term, immediate goals contribute to the patient's longer-term goals?

When you have completed this goal-setting exercise, consult the checklist in Table 2-2 where you will see listed some examples of good and poor interpersonal goals. Evaluate how likely your goal is to be achieved if you and the patient used it in social skills training.

STRUCTURED INSTRUMENTS FOR ASSESSING SOCIAL SKILLS

While no universally agreed-upon method has been developed to rate social skills and deficits of social skills, a variety of instruments have been used to get a "reading" on the patient's needs for training. The easiest to administer are questionnaires that the patient can fill out himself or herself prior to commencing social skills training. A number of such questionnaires have been published (see the Annotated Bibliography in the appendix), but one of the best validated is the Rathus Assertiveness Schedule. It is reprinted in Appendix D for readers who wish to use it in their clinical practice. This schedule, and others like it, taps such domains as avoiding social confrontation, being reluctant to express feelings and opinions, experiencing social anxiety and discomfort, making reasonable requests of others, refusing unreasonable requests of others, having problems in asserting one's rights, and expressing affection. Most inventories take into account the situational specificity of social skills deficits by including a wide range of affects and communications directed to a variety of significant others. After scoring a questionnaire such as this one, you can get some useful leads on the types of social and emotional situations that your patient may need training in. Before plunging into training, however, more focused and follow-up interviewing should be done.

Behavioral Interviewing

A focused interview, in which questions are asked to elicit and clarify the social transactions that are troublesome to a patient, can be a good way of gathering the raw material for subsequent training goals. Asking people what they would do (or have done) in actual situations may not reflect how they really perform in those situations, so interviews as well as other indirect methods of assessment may lack validity. However, if you have patients who can give a clear and graphic account of their social interactions, who are good observers of their own behavior, and who can report accurately on their interactions, a behavioral interview can be a fruitful initial assessment.

Prerequisites to a sound interview are relaxed rapport with the patient and clear orientation of the patient regarding the purpose and function of the questions and their answers. Questions need to be very specific so they can successfully elicit from the patient a description of the problematic communication or affective content, the people involved, the "where and when" of the situations, and the frequency of occurrences. Inquire also about the antecedents and consequences of particular problematic situations to gain a picture of behavioral sequences or events that "trigger" the situations, as well as their functional outcomes. For example, does the patient tend to invite criticism or aggression from others because of provocative behavior? Does the patient obtain needed sympathy or attention by experiencing social failures? Before skills training can be efficiently directed, the interpersonal context needs to be understood.

The kinds of questions asked in a full-scale interview are the same as those used during the goal-setting phase of social skills training.

- What types of difficulties do you have with others in your life?
- In which kinds of situations do these difficulties arise?
- What actually happens? Start from the beginning.
- How did you behave in that situation?
- How did the other person respond?
- Did you fail to attain your goals in that encounter?
- With whom did the problem occur?
- How often does this occur?

For example,

Therapist: What difficulties are you having in your life?
Patient: I have terrible back pain and I'm afraid I will have to quit my job.
Therapist: When you are working, when is the pain worse?
Patient: When my supervisor comes into my office with work assignments.
Therapist: What actually happens?
Patient: He usually asks me to work overtime or bring work home to do.
Therapist: Do you ever refuse?
Patient: No, because I don't want to make him angry.
Therapist: What happens when you accept the extra work?
Patient: I end up staying late or doing it at home, which interferes with my family life.
Therapist: Would you be willing to learn how to refuse unreasonable extra work politely or be able to negotiate with your supervisor about it?
Patient: Sure. But I get all choked up when this happens.
Therapist: I'll help you learn how to do it through social skills training.

In a structured behavioral interview, questions like these can focus on a spectrum of areas of interpersonal life, such as family interactions; work; shopping and commercial encounters dealing with social agencies; asserting one's rights; expressing anger, sadness, disappointment, annoyance, pleasure, and affection; recognizing and solving interpersonal problems; misinterpreting others' actions and feelings; and making requests of others to conform to one's desires.

Naturalistic Social Tests

While it is not usually possible to observe a patient's social behavior directly in the actual situations in which it freely and spontaneously occurs, confederates can be enlisted to structure and evaluate natural encounters. For example, let's see how Ted, introduced to you earlier in the text, is evaluated in a naturalistically styled test of his social skills deficits.

The therapist begins by orienting Ted to the test and obtaining his agreement to participate.

Therapist: Before we start social skills training, I'd like to evaluate your social skills by means of a simple and brief test. It'll only take five minutes. I'm going to introduce you to a stranger, who is a colleague of mine. I will ask him to present some challenges to your ability to carry on a conversation with him. To see how you handle these challenges, I'd like you to change the subject to sports at the first pause in the conversation. Ask him whether he likes baseball or football, and try to keep the topic on sports for a few minutes.

Ted: What if he doesn't like sports?

Therapist: Just try to find out why he doesn't. Or tell him about your interests in sports.

Ted: What else should I do?

Therapist: At the end of five minutes invite him to have a cup of coffee with you at the snackbar down the hall. I'll give you money to pay for the coffee. There'll be a clock on the wall that you can see.

Ted: That sounds OK.

Therapist: Then, after ten minutes have passed, break off the conversation and say goodbye.

Ted: It's a cinch.

Meantime, the confederate is given another set of instructions designed to apply mild social stress on Ted. The confederate is told to say, "I'm sorry, but I forgot your name," as soon as the therapist leaves the room. When Ted asks him for coffee, the confederate says firmly, "No thanks." When Ted terminates the conversation, the confederate asks him to give directions to a nonexistent building or bus stop. In this way, a patient can be assessed on how well he or she initiates and terminates a conversation and responds to some minor conversational challenges. Both the patient and the confederate fill out rating sheets that evaluate level of comfort, confidence, and competence during the ten-minute conversation.

Roleplay Assessments

Roleplay assessments are similar to confederate-based naturalistic tests, but they are designed to simulate real situations in a clinic, hospital, or private office. Since the setting can be carefully orchestrated, the roleplay test has the advantage of being easier to standardize, and the performance of the patient can be audiotaped or videotaped for later analysis. The disadvantage of the roleplay, however, is its obvious departure from reality, since the patient is aware that the evaluation is make believe. This means that a roleplay may engender less anxiety and be easier for a patient to perform than in real life. However, if a patient cannot perform reasonably well in the protected and safe environment of a "pretend it's real" roleplay, then it is unlikely that the patient can do so in real life. Thus, roleplay assessments tell clinicians more accurately about what patients *can't do* rather than what they can do.

Let's see how, Allen, whom we have already met, was evaluated in a roleplay test of his social skills relevant to his adaptation to a board-and-care home. A series of prototypical interpersonal situations, requiring both social initiative as well as assertive responses, is presented to Allen, and he is asked to respond to each one in turn. The situation includes being approached for conversation by a resident of the patient's board-and-care home, wanting to borrow something from a roommate, dealing with loud noise that is interfering with sleep, and trying to join a social gathering. This particular set of situations was selected as typical of the situations requiring social adjustment by patients living in a community-based residential care facility. A staff person rates appropriateness of Allen's verbal and nonverbal response to each situation. The form for the social skills roleplay is shown in Table 2-3.

Therapist: So that we can help new residents of our facility to improve their social skills, we conduct an assessment of how you respond to some typical situations you will encounter while you are living here.

Allen: I don't think I can do it. I'm no good at tests.

Therapist: There are no right or wrong answers. Even if you just sit and show no response at all, that will help us design a social skills training program for you. Just relax and try your best. I'll help you to respond to each situation by pretending that I'm the other person there with you. Watch my face and listen to what I say.

For the next few minutes, I am going to describe five different situations to you. I would like you to think about how you would respond to each situation and then act out what you would say or do. Let me show you what I mean. I will give a sample situation and act out how I would respond: My friend asks if he can borrow five dollars, and I don't have it. I say, "Gee, I'm sorry. I can't make a loan right now." Now I want you to try the same with the situations I am about to describe. Do you understand?

Allen: I think so. I'll try.

Therapist: Good. Here we go with the first situation. You are eating dinner in the dining room and another resident sits down next to you. You'd like to make some new friends, and he seems friendly. He says, "Hi. Dinner smells good, doesn't it?" Let's see how you respond to this situation, Allen.

Depending upon the patient's level of adjustment and the environment's social expectations, roleplay assessments can be designed to elicit information about the patient's capabilities in a variety of situations. For Allen and other residents of supervised community residential facilities, other roleplay situations could include the following:

- Being lost in the city and having to approach someone to ask directions.
- Asking a roommate to share some food or clothing item.

Table 2-3. Social Skills Roleplay Assessment.

This method of assessing social skills deficits is designed for seriously disabled mental patients living in residential care facilities. The assessor or social skills trainer poses each situation to the patient and asks the patient to act out how he or she might respond to the challenge inherent in the scenario. The test can be made to better simulate real-life settings by using props and by having the assessor, trainer, confederate, or another patient engage in an extended interaction during the scenario.

Score	Situations to Roleplay
_____	1. You are in the dining room and another resident sits next to you. You have wanted to get acquainted with this person and this is your chance.
_____	2. You are given an appointment to see a psychiatrist at a mental health center but you don't have any directions except the number of the bus to take. You catch the bus and have to find out how to get to the clinic.
_____	3. You have a tape cassette player and your roommate has a cassette that you would very much like to listen to. You've never borrowed anything from him in the past.
_____	4. You're trying to sleep after an exhausting day, but the TV is blaring very loudly in the next room. You know the residents who are watching TV, but sometimes they have been unfriendly to you. You also know the staff person on duty that night who has been helpful to you in the past.
_____	5. Several of your friends are talking together about going to a local restaurant for some coffee. You'd like to join them and walk up to where they are standing.

Scoring Key
   0 = behavior did not occur/was clearly inappropriate.
   1 = occurred minimally and did little to enhance communication/was marginally
      appropriate but requires improvement.
   2 = approached range of normal adult behavior.

Table 2-3. *Continued*

Definitions for Scoring Behaviors/Aspects

Behavior/Aspect	Appropriate	Inappropriate
Eye contact	Looks at other person Moves eyes while talking	Looks away from other Has fixed stare
Body posture	Body is erect while talking Appears relaxed	Slumps Very tense
Distance/physical contact	Stands a few feet away	Too close, too far Inappropriate touching
Gestures	Moves head and hands while talking	Stiff, no movement Exaggerated movements
Facial expressions	Smiles, frowns, wrinkles forehead, serious when necessary	Deadpan, no movement Expression matched to emotions
Voice inflection	Tone goes up and down with expression of feeling	Monotone, unusual inflection

Definitions for Scoring Behaviors/Aspects

Behavior/Aspect	Appropriate	Inappropriate
Latency of response	Responds without long pause Speaks at a moderate pace	Pauses for a long time Speaks too quickly or too slowly
Content of speech	Coherent, sensible, to the point	Loose associations, circum-stantial, tangential
Amount of speech	About right	Poverty of speech, mute, or excessive

Describe any behaviors that detracted from social performance (e.g., bizarre mannerisms) and record additional comments or observations _____

_____

_____

_____

Assessor _____

Date _____

- Requesting that a loaned item that's overdue be returned.
- Inviting a housemate to go out for a walk.
- Being bothered by another resident who's agitated and belligerent.
- Having a side effect of psychotropic medication and discussing it with the doctor.

The ratings from a social skills roleplay assessment can point the trainer or therapist in fruitful directions for goal setting as well as generate total scores that can be used to place the patient in a social skills training group appropriate to his or her overall level of social functioning. The roleplays can also be repeated after a period of training to document progress and give positive feedback to the patient. Alternatively, patients can be assigned to groups based upon their deficits in designated skill areas.

Permanent Products

An excellent and usually reliable way to assess patients' social competence is to examine the tangible products of their social transactions. With a clear rationale and explanation of the purpose, patients might be asked to divulge the contents of their wallet or purse since they could document the past occurrence of certain social experiences. For example, a library card and driver's license may be indicators of attendance at the public library and the motor vehicle agency. Business cards usually reflect contacts with the people and places inscribed on the card. Photos and an address book may indicate that the patient has friends and relatives still cherished and contacted. Identification and membership cards show affiliation with groups and organizations. Bank and credit cards may reflect a high level of capability in dealing with financial institutions.

Similarly, salary stubs can be used as evidence that a person has been successful in getting a job, purchased merchandise or receipts can reflect that the patient has been able to negotiate a shopping task, and theater stubs or restaurant match covers indicate that a recreational outing has been undertaken. Although this approach to assessment offers the advantage of being relatively unobtrusive and inexpensive in terms of time for the clinician, it suffers from the limitation of measuring only whether or not a task was performed successfully. More information, as elucidated by a behavioral interview, must be gathered to clarify what deficiencies led to unsuccessful outcomes. Permanent products are especially handy to confirm that a homework assignment was completed when monitoring patients' progress during social skills training.

In summing up the use of structured methods of assessing social skills, you should note that the available techniques offer a progression from most convenient to most cumbersome. Questionnaires and interviews are simple to use on the spot with a patient. Roleplay tests and naturalistic tests require time and effort to set the stage and instigate the patient and others to participate. While actually observing the patient in real life settings is the most valid type of assessment, it is also the most expensive and intrusive and is usually reserved for hospital situations where nursing staff can make the observations and report them to the therapist. If reliable relatives are willing and able, they can provide useful information regarding the patient's social behavior at home. Patients, themselves, can also observe their own actions and report them to the therapist. Each level of assessment presents increasing logistical difficulties, but yields a richer and more realistic harvest of assessment information.

SETTING THE STAGE

Before the goal setting is complete, you should obtain further details from the patient about the situation that will be practiced in the behavioral rehearsal. Details help to make the scene realistic, give everyone in the group a clear picture of what is to take place, and foster generalization to the real-life situation. Graphic descriptions of the setting, the people involved in the problem situation, and their actions and anticipated reactions make the session more like an enactment of the real situation. These concrete descriptions also enable patients to roleplay more easily and make the session more interesting and absorbing for those who are awaiting their turn to set goals and rehearse.

Short- and Long-Term Goals

Before launching into the dry run or initial rehearsal of an interpersonal situation, it is helpful to solicit from the patient his or her awareness of the immediate and longer-term goals inherent in the situation to be rehearsed. It is usually obvious to patients that they will be able to obtain some immediate need or desire by successful completion of the interaction being set up for roleplaying: However, the "forest is often lost sight of by preoccupation with the stress." For example, a patient who wants to get his or her doctor's cooperation in changing medication regimen may lose sight of the long-term goal, which is to establish and sustain a collaborative working relationship with the doctor. In the training process, care must be exercised to modulate the patient's performance and communications such that *both* the short-term and long-term goals are likely to be attained. In the example just given, it might be possible for the patient to hassle the doctor to the point that the doctor accedes to the patient's demands for a change in medication; however, this short-term success may come at the expense of the long-term doctor-patient relationship.

Having the patient deliberately and consciously consider both the long-term and short-term goals also confers a motivational benefit. When patients realize the more global and far-reaching consequences of attaining immediate interpersonal objectives, they can be primed to participate more actively in the social skills training steps and in carrying out their homework assignments. Consider the following patients who were helped to identify the long- and short-term goals for social skills training:

- Paul wanted to improve his grades in school. He chose to work on obtaining additional tutoring from his college instructor. His short-term goal was to gain the assent of the instructor for tutoring, and his longer-term goals were improved grades, graduation, and more independence from his parents from having better job prospects.
- George was having problems keeping within his minuscule income from Social Security. He decided to ask his doctor to prescribe nicotine-containing chewing gum so he could cut down on the costs of cigarettes. His short-term goal was to obtain a prescription for Nicorette chewing gum from his physician; his longer-term goals were to improve his health and have more disposable income to spend.
- Maureen wanted to break out of chronic social isolation, so she targeted conversations with strangers at volleyball games on the beach as a short-term goal. Her longer-term goal was eventually to meet people who would be candidates for enduring friendships.
- Mel was disabled with multiple sclerosis as well as suffering from chronic depression and alcoholism. He opted to make phone calls to service organizations to locate a person who would be willing to provide transportation for him to get around town to attend social activities. Longer-term goals related to his wanting to find a woman with whom he could have a romantic and intimate relationship.

Use Behavioral Rehearsal for "On-Line" Assessment

When it is not clear how the targeted other person in the situation might react to the patient's communication, or if you and the patient think the reaction might be cold, rejecting, or indifferent, it is advisable to develop a series of situations for the subsequent rolepaly, each with the roleplayer expressing more and more unpleasant responses "scripted" for the target person. It's important to start with a receptive response to give the patient some initial reinforcement for efforts, but as repeated practice consolidates the skill for the patient, increments of negative affect can be incorporated by the roleplayer in response to the patient. For example, in the goal setting described for Ted, the person roleplaying his supervisor, Mr. Houk, could in successive rehearsals move from friendly to more and more hostile reactions to Ted.

Because some people try to talk a scene to death instead of practicing, the counselor or leader must provide flexible guidance in eliciting the "who?" "what?" "when?" "where?" and "how?" of the scene or situation. Forget the "why?" and guide the participant toward specific portrayal of some recent example of the problem situation, or an example in the near future. Avoid listening or probing for reasons why the participant has difficulty with the emotions, communication, and people depicted in the scene. Speculation on motives only leads to boredom and endless talk, deterring the patient and the leader from moving on to remedial action.

Remember, the task is to get to the point quickly. Get the scene on, get it off, and do it again. Specifics, action, and repetition are the soul of learning. Don't get bogged down in redundant details, but get the patient to provide enough background information to make the scene real. Choose situations for rehearsal that occur often in the person's life. Then find out if the situation requires the roleplayers to stand up or sit down, or if the scene requires a surrogate who is old or young, or if some props might be helpful, such as in the case of playing a scene where the participant is returning defective merchandise to a store.

Encouraging participants to set the stage with graphic details make them feel that they are helping to plan and manage the treatment process. The mystique of psychotherapy is abandoned by involving the clients as active agents in their own therapy. The counselor assists the patient in selecting and developing good scenes to practice without wasting valuable time on trivial or harmful behavioral goals.

Once the scene is described properly, the patient picks another member of the group to serve as a surrogate for the role of the person in real life with whom he or she wants to improve communication or emotional expression. If the roleplayed situation involves several people, the participant and the leader call upon several members of the group to enact the scene. When choosing surrogate roleplayers, the patient and the leader are guided by the similarity rule: the surrogates should have similar characteristics to the real-life individuals they are portraying. Characteristics of importance in establishing realism include age, sex, nonverbal behaviors, assertiveness, and communication style. Surrogates can be chosen as models of the actual people from among the staff or patients.

The surrogate needs to know the characteristics of the person whose role is being taken so that appearance and response style can be satisfactorily mimicked. If the surrogate is the patient's husband, who is middle-aged and overbearing, then a middle-aged man should be chosen and told how to act by the patient and the leader. While surrogates for roleplaying can be solicited through volunteers, the leader will many times find active selection more expedient and less anxiety provoking. The leader also will be in a better position to move the group into action with prompts, modeling, and feedback if he or she is standing up and moving around the room. Leadership in social skills training requires an active, "out-of-the-seat," active therapist or counselor.

Using other members of the group as surrogates for "interpersonal targets" produces a hidden bonus for social learning. The people taking others' roles practice a range of characters and behaviors. This loosens inhibitions and provides opportunities to gain experiences with new and different response styles. Also, when a particular, significant other person is not involved in the problem situation, a useful strategy is to replay the same situation several times using different surrogates as roleplayers. This approach fosters flexibility. The patient, learning social skills by reacting to different kinds of "interpersonal targets," has a chance to try a variety of responses and styles, thereby building a broader behavioral repertoire. Practicing with a number of dissimilar roleplayers facilitates generalization of the newly learned social skills to the real world, where the unpredictability of everyday life sometimes produces reactions that were not anticipated during the behavioral rehearsal. To summarize,

1. Describe in detail what is to take place in the scene—the "who?" "what?" "when?" "where?" and "how?" of the problem situation.
2. Provide flexible guidance when supporting the patient's active participation in choosing a scene and setting the stage for the scene.
3. Use roleplayers who have characteristics similar to those with whom the patient will interact in the real-life situation.
4. Use a number of roleplayers reflecting different response styles when teaching skills that are not being applied to a specific, significant other person.

Here is an example of a scene being set up by a therapist for a patient, Charles, who complained of problems on his job. Part of Charles's problem resulted from his reluctance to ask his boss questions; consequently, he made many mistakes, which caused his boss to become irritable with him and which, in turn made Charles even more afraid to ask questions.

Therapist: OK, Charles, we are going to work on the problem you have asking your boss to repeat the instructions he gives you. With whom would you like to work?

Charles: Maria.

Therapist: Is your boss a woman, Charles?

Charles: No, a man.

Therapist: Well why don't you work with a man, then, since it will be easier to pretend that it's actually your boss. Who in the group reminds you most of your boss?

Charles: Tom does.

Therapist: Would you help Charles by roleplaying his boss, Tom?

Tom: Sure.

Therapist: Charles, tell Tom how your boss acts when he gives instructions. How does he talk and what does he say?

Charles: Well, he talks real loud so it's hard to interrupt him, and he talks fast, too. Sometimes he paces back and forth.

Therapist: Charles, you told us that your boss gave you some instructions last week regarding the time schedule of some shipments. You really didn't get it straight, but you didn't ask him to repeat it. Would you like to try that scene now with Tom?

Charles: Can I also practice complaining to him about talking so fast when he gives directions?

Therapist: Maybe we can work on that later, but for now let's just work on improving your grasp of his instructions to you. Whether he talks too fast or too slow, you still have to learn how to get the instructions straight. Tom, do you understand the situation? Give Charles a time schedule for some shipments. For instance, "Send out the Rochester shipment at 2:30, the Cleveland shipment at 3:50, and so on." When you play the scene, talk loud and fast and pace back and forth a little, too. OK?

Tom: OK.

Therapist: Charles, I want to see how you handle this situation where Tom is taking the part of your boss at the point where you lose track of the instructions. Show us what usually happens.

Notice that the therapist went over each of the following points.

1. He suggested that a male surrogate roleplay the boss since Charles's boss is male.
2. He promoted a detailed description of the scene for all participants.
3. He guided the choice of the scene when the patient suggested a more difficult one.
4. He elicited the response style of the roleplayed figure to make the performance more realistic.

Here is one more example with a patient, Norma, who complained of a lack of privacy in her life. Her therapist questioned her about this and found out that part of Norma's problem was caused by one of her neighbors, who frequently used her telephone.

Therapist: Let's try that scene with your neighbor today, Norma, OK? You said that you'd like to learn how to go about suggesting that she get her own phone. Who would you like to work with?

Norma: Annette.

Therapist: Fine, Annette, would you like to roleplay Norma's neighbor?

Annette: Sure. What should I do?

Therapist: Norma has mentioned that her neighbor knocks on her door and asks to use her phone. Basically, that's what you'll do. Norma, can you tell us a little more about how your neighbor acts, and what she says when she comes to use your phone?

Norma: She usually walks right in before I even ask her in; then she starts dialing the phone while she's asking me if she can use it.

Therapist: What does she usually say?

Norma: She usually has some "urgent" reason to use the phone, but the calls don't sound that important to me.

Therapist: How does she act when she comes in?

Norma: She starts talking very fast about the call as soon as I open the door, then she just about runs to the phone and dials before I can say anything. By the time I can open my mouth she's already talking on the phone.

Therapist: Annette, do you understand what to do?

Annette: Yes, I knock on the door and use the phone.

Therapist: Right. But also act like you're in a hurry. Talk fast and walk quickly to the phone, talking all the time. Tell Norma that the call is about something very important.

Annette: OK. I can do that.

Therapist: Good. Norma, when Annette starts walking in, use hand gestures to indicate that you want her to "wait a minute." Don't be afraid to interrupt her and ask her exactly why she has to use the phone. Stop her from dialing if you have to. Remember, you want to talk to her about the phone calls, and you have to interrupt her before she makes the call.

Norma: What should I say to her?

Therapist: We can work on that later. For now just practice how it has gone with her in the past. We'll watch for what you do well and what can be improved.

PRACTICE EXERCISE

From among your current cases, select one patient with an affiliative skill deficit. Pinpoint a specific interpersonal situation that reflects the patient's deficits and elaborate the scene that might serve as a starting point for social skills training. Be sure to indicate what the patient's short- and long-term goals are in the situation and where, when, and with whom the interaction is to take place. Use the stepwise procedures for assessment of social skills shown in Table 2-4 to develop appropriate goals and situations for skills training.

(continued)

Remind your patient that being socially skillful does not require smooth and slick responses, but rather making an effort with some reasonable amount of coaching from a therapist. There are many different ways to express one's feelings and obtain one's needs— trial and error will eventually lead to successful experiences. Persistence is encouraged and learning from one's experiences requires time and effort.

SUMMARY

Because social skills training is nonspecific, there are no special kinds of patients or problems for which the technique cannot be useful. Only those patients who can't pay attention and follow simple instructions for 15 minutes are not considered ready for social skills training. Incoherence and thought disorder as well as acute agitation and emotional turmoil are the primary causes of poor attentional ability. Severe short-term memory problems, seen in organic mental disorders, can also make this type of training difficult and fatiguing. In general, trying the patient in a training session will be the most informative test of how appropriately the patient will behave in social skills training.

The most important part of social skills training occurs before any training sessions start: Assessment of the patient's existing skills and deficits and the choice of long- and short-term goals. Assessment and training are closely linked in social skills training. Use direct observation of how the patient behaves in simulated social situations, along with the usual methods of acquiring assessment information about patients. Past treatment records; interviews with the patient, family, friend and acquaintances; and questionnaires or rating scales should all be employed to discover the existing skills, prominent deficits and the social situations that are critical to the patient's adjustment. Even if there is little to go on in the way of records and background, the patient can be exposed to a training session virtually "cold" since a wealth of important information will be quickly developed. In fact, a drop-in therapy group called "Successful Living" that relies heavily on social skills assessment and training has been helpful to a diverse range of psychiatric patients, some of whom only come once or twice for crisis intervention.

Social skills can be sorted into instrumental skills and affiliative skills. Instrumental skills are used in social interactions centered around work and service relationships. They help patients learn things that are needed to survive in community life. Affiliative or social-emotional skills, are employed to acquire, deepen, and maintain friendships and family relationships. Instrumental and affiliative skills should meet eight criteria before being used as goals in training. Skills targeted as goals should be (1) attainable, (2) positive and constructive behaviors, (3) specific, (4) functional, (5) consistent with the patient's rights and responsibilities, (6) chosen by the patient, (7) high-frequency behaviors, and (8) likely to occur in the near future.

As you zero in to set the highly specific goals required by social skills training, you will have to use very pointed questions. This will have the effect of diverting the patients' attention away from their symptoms and

Table 2-4. Social Skills Assessment by the Numbers

Step	Procedure
1. Determine ability of patient to follow instructions, pay attention.	Rule out severe incoherence and conceptual disorganization in schizophrenic or organic disorders. Use lowest effective dosage of psychotropics. Try structured activity to displace intrusive and bizarre symptoms.
2. Do initial assessment of patient's social skills before starting training.	Checklist of criteria in Table 2-2. Examine histories and assessments in medical record. Talk to caregivers, family, responsible clinicians. Use results of assessment instruments. Observe patient yourself.
3. Evaluate patient's affiliative and instrumental abilities.	Set up "dry run" with two or three helpers (staff or other patients). Help patient put problems in interpersonal context.
4. Check stressors in patient's life: time-limited events, ongoing tensions, conflicts.	Look for big changes, overstimulation, overinvolvement of family, caregiver, drugs, alcohol use.
5. Check coping skills.	Ask what changes patient would make, what situations make for lack of confidence, social anxiety. See if there are constructive activities that patient can engage in to displace symptoms.
6. Identify tentative goals and scenes for roleplaying and training.	Involve patient as much as possible and use all other sources of assessment data.
7. Use structured instruments for further assessment.	Focused behavioral interview. Do naturalistic observation. Do roleplay test. Examine permanent products of patient's social life.
8. Obtain as many details as possible for the scenes you will use first.	Ask "who?" "what?" "where?" "when?" and "how often?" Get descriptions of physical setting, people, and events.
9. Be sure goals are positive, attainable, specific functional, high frequency, consistent with rights, responsibilities, chosen by patient as likely to occur.	Use these criteria to be sure the goals, situations will be useful and productive in training.

toward more functional goal setting. Identifying and describing the patients' stressors and available coping skills in detail are essential for the goal-setting process. Stressors are of two types: time-limited life events that have a definite beginning and end, and ambient tensions and conflicts that arise from ongoing relationships with other people. While the former are usually easy to uncover, the latter often require more inquiry. Patients who experience overprotectiveness, emotional overinvolvement or excessive criticism on a day-to-day basis are far more likely to relapse. Too much social support may be a dangerous thing! Goals that displace symptoms or divert attention from general complaints are very useful in raising morale and the expectations of patients.

While there are scales and inventories that are applicable to goal setting for social skills, we prefer focused, behavioral interviews. Eliciting detailed descriptions of patients' own behavior in the context of the social situations they encounter can be very helpful in developing goals. Some unorthodox methods can and should be used in assessment: Naturalistic social tests using confederates, roleplay rehearsals, and examination of permanent products from behavioral assignments can yield convergent and reliable information about the way patients respond to their social worlds.

Chapter 3
Training Social Skills

Now that an initial functional or behavioral assessment has been described for patients in need of social skills training, we can begin to describe the steps used in the training. While initial assessments can be very helpful in determining areas of deficiency and need, more specific assessment continues to be carried out during the training process itself. In fact, ongoing assessment is tightly interwoven with the training steps and serves to provide guidance and feedback to the trainer in pacing the training and in selecting continuing goals and scenes. For example, in the "dry run" or first behavioral rehearsal of the training sequence, you will directly observe how deficient or skillful your patient actually is while he or she rehearses.

It is also important to conceptualize social skills training in a larger context—the comprehensive range of services and treatment that most severely mentally ill persons require. As can be seen in Figure 3-1, skills training is but one element in an array of treatment modalities and community support services needed by patients with chronic mental disorders—all keyed to the stage of an individual's illness. Most chronic and seriously mentally ill persons need pharmacological treatment, crisis intervention, family therapy, medical care, inpatient and day hospital care, vocational rehabilitation, and other treatment services. As shown in Table 3-1, these services must be available indefinitely through a responsible agency or mental health center that provides case management and *continuity of care*. By promoting greater independence, social skills training may reduce the total amount of these services required by patients over the long haul.

In this chapter, we shall describe in graphic detail the step-by-step procedure of training social skills, using a model that includes the necessity of teaching patients skills in social perception and problem solving. These perceptual and cognitive skills are essential if patients are to be

The "Complex Cube" of Psychiatric Rehabilitation

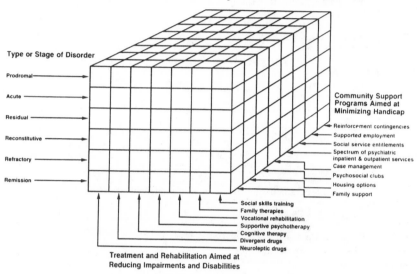

FIGURE 3-1. The complex cube of psychiatric rehabilitation shows the three dimensions that need to be covered in a comprehensive approach to providing services to the seriously mentally disabled. Social skills training is but one element of treatment that is imbedded in a broader network of services and keyed to the stage of a person's disorder. For example, social skills training should not be given to patients in the throes of acute psychotic symptoms but should be reserved for later stages of the illness, as symptoms subside.

able to select and use effective communications that are appropriate to the interpersonal situations they must face.

This social skills model harnesses all the techniques and principles that have been found to promote human learning. As shown in Table 3-2, these principles include abundant positive reinforcement for even small signs of improvement or effort—something that the therapist must do, even if it seems at times to be patronizing. Keep in mind that most patients with serious mental illnesses have had little positive feedback

Table 3-1. The Multiple Facets of a Comprehensive, Community-Based Mental Health Service for the Chronically Mentally Ill. Each facet must be available to patients and their caregivers if social skills training is to be maximally effective, durable, and generalizable.

1. Responsible, "lead" agency
   Accountable
   Accessible
   Coordination
   Case management and outreach

2. Spectrum of psychiatric therapies
   Full and partial hospitalization
   Pharmacotherapy
   Crisis and emergency intervention
   Skills training
   Psychosocial clubs and self-help groups
   Supportive psychotherapy
   Family interventions

3. Range of social and medical services

   | Medical | Legal | Vocational |
   | Financial | Housing | Advocacy |

4. Flexible levels of intervention
   Individualized assessment and treatment that is available indefinitely

5. Treatment and rehabilitation offered
   In vivo (natural settings)
   Twenty-four hours a day
   With a positive, "can do" attitude

Table 3-2. Principles of Learning That Are Mobilized for Use in the Structuring and Process of Social Skills Training

- Individualized specification and targeting problems and goals in behavioral and operational terms
- Measurement and monitoring of behavioral progress
- Functional analysis of environmental antecedents and consequences that may be maintaining behavioral problems and deficits
- Identifying reinforcers that can serve to motivate participation and progress
- Compensating for cognitive deficits by use of audiovisual and other media
- Optimal types and doses of psychotropic drugs that promote, not impede, learning
- Reinforcement of small increments of adaptive behavior (shaping)
- Therapeutic instructions and expectancy
- Social modeling—"live" and video
- Repeated practice and overlearning
- Active prompting and coaching
- Positive feedback for progress
- Generalization to real-life settings

for their learning efforts in the past and have considerable cognitive and attitudinal problems that add up to a "learning disability." To overcome these disabilities, social skills training resembles a special education classroom rather than a conventional, insight-oriented therapy session.

TRAINING SOCIAL SKILLS IN GROUPS

While this chapter will describe social skills training procedures for use in a group format, the very same stepwise method can be applied to individual therapy, couples therapy, and family therapy. In fact, some of the best documented examples of the efficacy of social skills training have been produced by researchers working one-on-one, in marital therapy sessions and in family therapy. Our use of social skills training in groups stems from the considerable cost-effectiveness available from conducting psychosocial interventions in groups as well as the added opportunities for learning from one's peers through multiple role models, group cohesion, and reinforcement. The advantages of conducting social skills training in groups are listed in Table 3-3.

When new patients enter a group they quickly develop positive expectations for treatment by witnessing the progress reported and exhibited by veteran group members. Likewise, patients making slower progress and having greater behavioral deficits can learn from and be encouraged by observing the improvement shown by others. Practicing communica-

Table 3-3. Advantages of Training Social Skills in Group Format

1. A group, with its ready availability of social interaction among members, provides multiple, naturalistic, and spontaneous opportunities for practicing skills.
2. The group arena offers a forum for the therapist to frequently assess patients informally exhibiting their social skills, reflecting progress in training.
3. Reinforcement of learned skills is amplified by peer feedback, in addition to therapist feedback, and may be more credible than feedback from therapist.
4. Modeling options are multiplied by availability of peers who can provide more realistic and congruent models for a patient than a therapist.
5. Patients can serve as "buddies" for each other in facilitating the completion of homework assignments.
6. Motivation to persevere in skills training is enhanced by the presence of more advanced, "veteran" patients whose progress can encourage "beginners."
7. Orientation and favorable expectations for "new" patients can be given by "veteran" patients in a way that adds to the impact of the therapist.
8. Group cohesion magnifies the positive influence on symptomatic relief that derives from the therapeutic relationship.
9. Group training is more efficient than individual training as four to eight patients can be led by a single therapist.

tion skills in a group also facilitates the generalization of rehearsed behaviors to real-life situations. The group setting bears similarities to many situations in everyday life, where the individual has opportunities to practice expressing feelings and making social contacts. Generalization of newly learned behaviors to novel situations is enhanced by tailoring the group training sessions to resemble actual situations the person will encounter in real life. While the presence of a group may initially inhibit some patients' participation, it is also true that moderately stressful conditions for learning more closely resemble the stressors found in real-life conditions. If a person can do well in a social skills training group, there is a better chance that he or she will also do well in natural, family, social, and work groups. Rather than creating a learning environment that is a haven from the real world, social skills training emphasizes real-life situations and their mastery through speech and action.

Social skills training is carried out in groups of 4 to 10 patients preferably with two professional or paraprofessional leaders. Individual training sessions, between one patient and a therapist or counselor, can also be used as a supplement to group sessions. Social skills groups are often conducted with a group of individuals who have needs in a common area, such as conversational skills or the ability to develop recreational activities. Patients participating in such groups need not have the same level of functioning, although some commonality in skill deficits is assumed. However, social skills groups can also be conducted with patients who do not share deficits in the same skills. With heterogeneous groups, interpersonal problem areas are identified for the various patients, and specific skills are targeted for training based on the needs and goals of each individual patient.

If your institution, agency, or practice is large enough, you may have sufficient patients to assign to separate groups organized to help teach methods for coping with relatively demarcated problems, such as anxiety, depression, marital problems, and difficulty in assertion. Inpatient and day treatment social skills groups are often organized to address specific problem areas common to psychiatric patients, such as basic conversational skills, inability to express positive and negative feelings, lack of self-care and grooming, a dearth of recreational activities, the need for vocational adjustment and job interviewing skills, and the lack of friendship and dating skills. In Table 3-4 are listed common problem areas and the social skills taught in a typical community mental health center.

Group training sessions generally last between 45 and 90 minutes and can be conducted as infrequently as once a week or as often as once a

Table 3-4. Social and Independent Living Skills Taught to Outpatients and Day Care Patients in a Community Mental Health Center

Problem Areas	Skills Training Groups
Initiating and maintaining conversations	Basic, intermediate, and advanced conversational skills
Dating and friendships	Dating and friendship skills
Budgeting and consumerism	Money management skills
Assertive use of social services and entitlement	Public agencies
Marital discord	Marital communication skills
Family stress and conflict	Family communication and problem solving
Child behavior problems	Parent training group
Unemployment	Job finding skills
Indolence with leisure time	Recreation for leisure group
Personal hygiene problems	Grooming and self-care skills
Medication noncompliance	Medication self-management
Relapses	Symptom self-management
Crises	Successful living group
Anxiety and depression	Stress management group
Aggression and hostility	Anger management training

day. Patients suffering from chronic psychiatric illnesses, such as schizophrenia, major depression, manic-depression, and severe personality disorders, require more intensive social skills training because of the duration and extent of their social disabilities and cognitive and attentional deficits; in fact, frequent training sessions and between-session practices are necessary for severely impaired patients. Closely spacing the group sessions facilitates more rapid acquisition and generalization of the relevant social skills. *Overlearning* skills, by repeatedly practicing them beyond the point of the first few successes, is advantageous since it promotes durability of the skills and their transfer to novel situations.

STRUCTURING AND PACING A SOCIAL SKILLS SESSION

As you move into the actual social skills session, you may feel you've suddenly gotten into theater work or sports rather than the serious business of helping people get along better in this world. We do emphasize behavioral rehearsal, and at times you may feel like a stage director or sports coach rather than a therapist or a counselor. But remember, the purpose of social skills training is to teach patients to communicate their needs and feelings to others in a positive, productive manner, and the best way we know to be sure that people learn is to have them practice the real situation again and again. Repeated practice is essential. The emphasis is on rehearsal, and just as actors in theaters and players on the field learn from the feedback they get from the director or coach, our own patients learn by the feedback they get from us and from their fellow patients.

There is one big difference between the actor preparing for a performance and our patients preparing for their performances. The actor will still perform in a make-believe situation—even if it is before an audience. Our patients will perform in real life, and for them there is high drama in the most common situations.

In this chapter we'll cover the mechanics of running a social skills training session. We've found that a little structure goes a long way, and we've developed a number of strategies and shortcuts that should make your job easier and more enjoyable. The method developed over a period of many years, as well as the exercises and the theatrical or athletic terms, were adopted because they enhanced cohesion, streamlined the process, and promoted learning and the patients seemed to enjoy them. The pace of training was deliberately heightened to maintain everyone's interest and to allow the therapists to teach skills to everyone in the group.

This structuring and pacing of the sessions was motivated by more than just a desire to finish sessions on time. Very early we found that people—both patients *and* therapists—had a tendency to talk a lot about the whys and wherefores of the problems, symptoms, and complexities present in any situation. Speculation on psychodynamics and motives, "war stories" of various kinds, rationalizations, alibis, and other irrelevancies kept intruding and getting in the way of actually *doing* something. Whether motivated by anxiety or just the well-known tendency of those in mental health to worry a problem to death, we found that such talk reduced the number of times a person could practice and get feedback. Be wary of this trap. When it occurs, patients and therapists alike get restless, fall asleep, or otherwise become inattentive. If you ever find yourself bored in social skills training, it's probably because the action has been brought to a grinding halt by someone talking too much and not doing anything. We call this the MEGO syndrome: "Mine Eyes Glaze Over." Break it up—in a socially acceptable way, of course—and get back on track.

Naturally, after you've had some practice, you will add your own embellishments and personal style of leadership. The basic structure is there only to ensure that you cover all the important parts of the training. By going through the training very systematically, both patients and therapists come to have high expectations of one another. If a step is skipped, patients will interrupt to tell you about it. And that's a good sign that they are paying attention. Done properly, it's hard for patients not to pay attention in these sessions.

One last suggestion about keeping everyone's attention: Stay on your feet! Most mental health professionals are used to conducting therapy sessions from a chair, and this on-your-feet style may be a bit uncomfortable at first. But unless you are involved in a practice situation that calls for you to be sitting down, stand up and be ready to position yourself close to the action. It's not necessary for the co-therapist to stand while waiting to work with patients, but whoever is directing the action should avoid doing it from a chair.

This is more than just a moralistic admonition—it is a very practical suggestion. You have to keep moving around to be able to see what people are really doing as they practice; to be able to provide them with encouraging prompts and praise, you have to be mobile. When you ask for feedback from other group members you should move closer to them. Move freely around the room, gesture broadly, speak more loudly than you usually do, and be very appreciative and demonstrative of any positive contribution. If this seems to be exaggerated and overly dramatic, it is meant to be. Patients with major mental disorders are frequently inhibited and inactive or distracted; so, keeping patients' attention focused on learning skills through the action of the session requires vigilance and creativity. Be a good model for patients to imitate. Move around and don't be afraid to be energetic, expressive, and even charismatic. The overall atmosphere should be upbeat—something between an elementary school classroom and a revival meeting.

Setting the Stage for Social Skills Training

Let's go through a social skills training session as offered in a group format. Between 4 and 10 patients is a good size group for social skills training. Up to 15 can be included, but a second therapist is essential to run the session since larger groups can make for long, tiring sessions. If you have the option of having a co-therapist for all your sessions, we would recommend you do so. Social skills training is demanding, and it's good to have another person helping by alternatively working with individual patients, keeping records, and making out assignment cards. If video equipment is being used, the co-therapist can operate the camera and recorder.

Because remembering all the important details in a social interaction of only 20 or 30 seconds can be frustrating, video feedback is very effective. The television camera captures it all. Fortunately, with today's sophisticated, relatively inexpensive equipment, video feedback can be used fairly smoothly in a social skills session. There are some cautions, however. One is the fact that the television system, and not the patient, can become the focus of the session. Fiddling with the camera, rewinding the tape to just the right place, fast-forwarding, and searching can become a distraction that slows the pace and bores the audience. Second, the monitor should be large enough for everyone to see clearly. Third, the sound system of most inexpensive systems is marginal, so you may have to work with a high-quality microphone remote from the camera. Last, too many wires can restrict movement and spontaneity. If you can overcome these potential problems, and employ the video as an adjunct rather than the main source of feedback, by all means do so. And remember, the video feedback shown to your patients will enhance the acquisition of skills only if they are exposed to their *improved* performances. Do not succumb to the tendency to reveal and confront patients with their deficits or inappropriate social behavior.

The room should be comfortable and large enough to allow people to move around easily. It should be well lit and ventilated, and a no-smoking policy should be in effect, except during break times. There is no necessity for props, although common items can be used to make the roleplays seem more realistic. If a spare, unplugged telephone is available, it can be used often in the behavioral rehearsals. Pencil and paper help to simulate an office setting, and a newspaper helps in scenes where someone has to get another person's attention.

A blackboard or easel with newsprint pads should be available, since you will want to document the specific behavioral targets for training through the visual as well as audio channel. Ratings can also be made on a flipchart or blackboard that give positive feedback to patients as they improve during the action. Make some posters to display on the walls of the room during the sessions (see Figures 3-2 to 3-5). They will serve as handy cues and prompts for patients and therapists. A clipboard can be used for recording patients' progress. Examples of progress notes suitable for insertion into the medical record are included in the Appendix to this guidebook. A package of $3'' \times 5''$ cards will also be handy for writing homework assignments. In Figure 3-6 is shown one type of card that has been used effectively for many years of training psychiatric patients. Assignment cards can be printed up ahead of time and given to patients as a reminder. Other than these few extras, no special equipment is necessary.

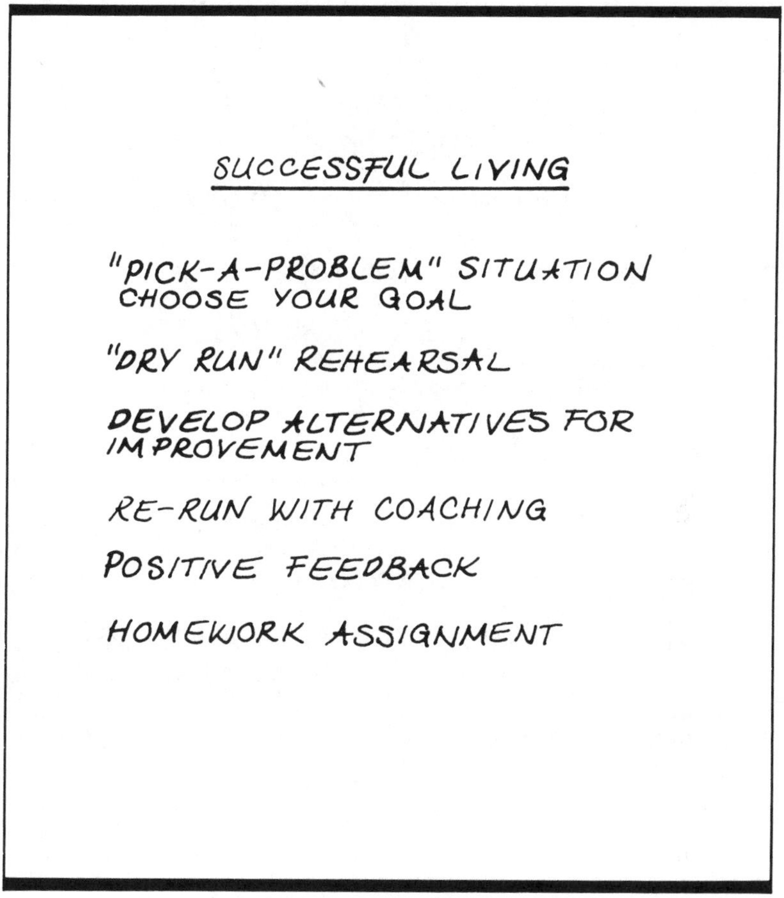

SUCCESSFUL LIVING

"PICK-A-PROBLEM" SITUATION
CHOOSE YOUR GOAL

"DRY RUN" REHEARSAL

DEVELOP ALTERNATIVES FOR
IMPROVEMENT

RE-RUN WITH COACHING

POSITIVE FEEDBACK

HOMEWORK ASSIGNMENT

FIGURE 3-2. Charts can be used to good advantage in a social skills training session to cue patients and therapists alike in adhering to the structural procedure. In this chart, the steps of basic training are listed from goal setting to homework assignments.

OPENING A GROUP SOCIAL SKILLS TRAINING SESSION: ORIENTATION AND SETTING FAVORABLE EXPECTATIONS

A handy map to guide your structuring a social skills training session is shown in Table 3-5. This map will take you, step by step, through a basic social skills training session and can be relied upon to give good results. The first six steps are covered in this section of the chapter, although the tasks required to build useful interpersonal scenes for train-

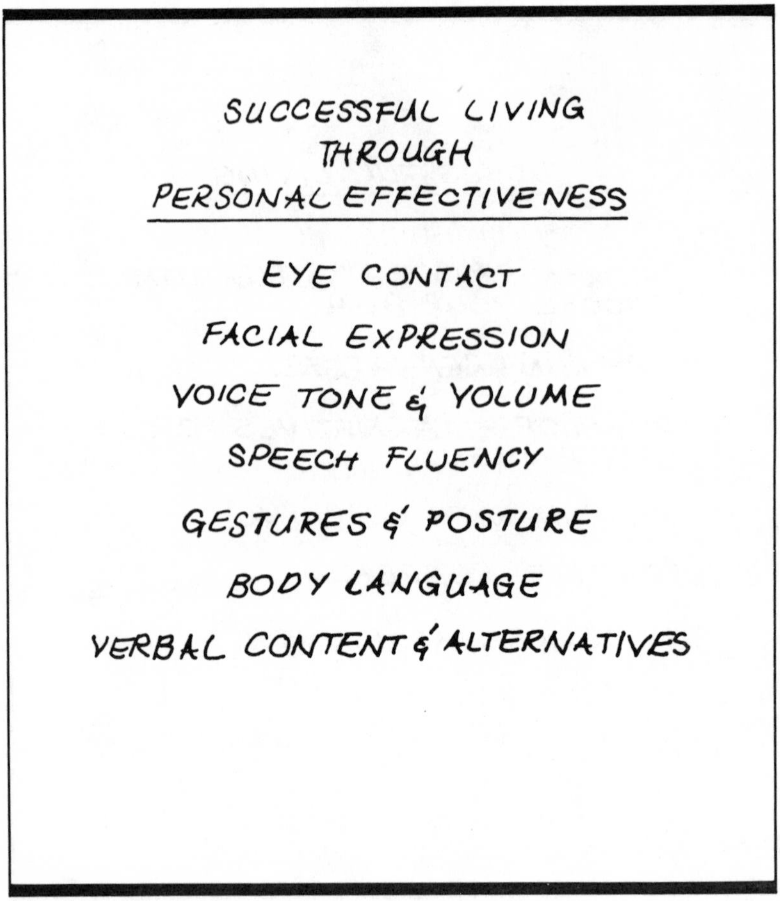

SUCCESSFUL LIVING
THROUGH
PERSONAL EFFECTIVENESS

EYE CONTACT

FACIAL EXPRESSION

VOICE TONE & VOLUME

SPEECH FLUENCY

GESTURES & POSTURE

BODY LANGUAGE

VERBAL CONTENT & ALTERNATIVES

FIGURE 3-3. The verbal, paralinguistic, and nonverbal elements of social skills are shown in this poster, which is used in an open-ended training group that is called, Successful Living Through Personal Effectiveness.

ing were also covered in detail in Chapter 2, "Assessing Social Skills." This map or guide for trainers will be reprinted in subsequent sections of this chapter, highlighting the relevant steps to be taken as you move through a typical session.

The first part of every session is used for introducing new patients, when running an open group, and in getting reports on how well patients did on their assignments from the last session. The introduction of new patients is valuable for new and "old" patients because it also serves as a good review of the purposes of social skills training for everyone. The therapist prompts the "old" patients to give most of the explanation

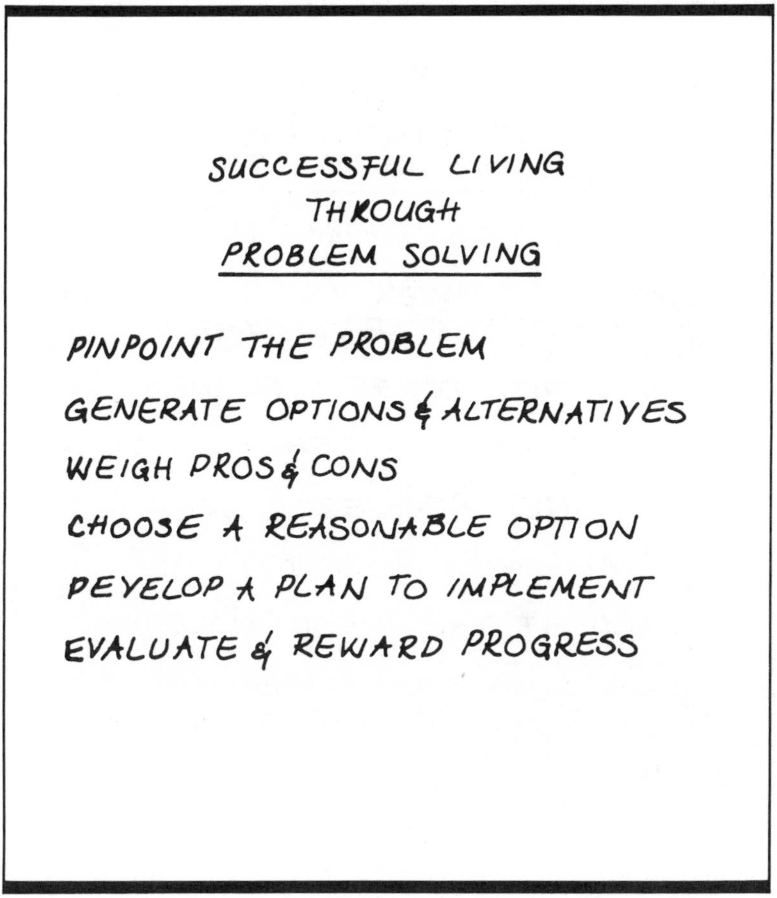

SUCCESSFUL LIVING
THROUGH
PROBLEM SOLVING

PINPOINT THE PROBLEM

GENERATE OPTIONS & ALTERNATIVES

WEIGH PROS & CONS

CHOOSE A REASONABLE OPTION

DEVELOP A PLAN TO IMPLEMENT

EVALUATE & REWARD PROGRESS

FIGURE 3-4. The steps for doing social problem-solving are shown in this chart, also mounted on the wall of the room in which the Successful Living group meets.

of the goals and methods for orienting new patients to the format of the session. So the new patient learns from fellow patients, who really serve as models for progress and hope as well as give information. The therapist learns how well the patients have learned to conceptualize the purpose of social skills training, getting another kind of feedback on how effective the training has been. It is also advisable to provide new patients with orientation to the rationale and procedure of social skills training before they attend their first group meeting. This can be done efficiently by distributing a descriptive brochure such as the one printed in the Appendix to this guidebook. You may want to photocopy this

SUCCESSFUL LIVING

ALTERNATIVES FOR SOLVING PROBLEMS

TERMINATE OR WITHDRAW POLITELY.

COME BACK LATER ASK FOR A DELAY OR MAKE LATER APPOINTMENT.

COMPLY WITH OTHER'S REQUEST.

REPEAT YOUR REQUEST POSITIVELY.

MAKE A NEW REQUEST.

EXPLAIN YOUR POSITION.

HIGHLIGHT THE IMPORTANCE OF YOUR NEEDS.

ASK FOR ASSISTANCE OR HELP.

COMPROMISE.

IGNORE CRITICISM.

ACKNOWLEDGE POSITIVES WITH THANKS.

GIVE COMPLIMENTS OR PRAISE

FIGURE 3-5. In guiding patients through social problem solving, it is helpful to refer to the generic types of alternatives or options that can be utilized by patients as they face situations that challenge them to achieve their short-term and long-term goals. This chart, used in the Successful Living group, is kept on the wall during the training sessions and serves to cue patients and trainers as they attempt to generate alternatives to solving problems.

SOCIAL SKILLS TRAINING
ASSIGNMENT - REPORT CARD

Name _____

Date assignment given _____

Assignment _____

_____

Date assignment due _____(_____)

(check when completed)

                    Therapist's initials _____

(front)

CUES FOR PERSONAL EFFECTIVENESS

1. Maintain **EYE CONTACT**

2. Use your **HANDS**

3. Lean **TOWARD** the other person

4. Pleasant **FACIAL EXPRESSION**

5. Speak with **FIRM TONE** and **FLUENT** pace

(back)

FIGURE 3-6. An example of the front and back of a 3″×5″ assignment card given to patients to remind them of their homework assignments from the social skills training session.

Table 3-5. Step-by-Step Map for Guiding Therapists Through a Typical Session of Social Skills Training

What to Do	How to Do It
1. Give introduction to social skills training.	Welcome patients, introduce yourself, give a brief description of the purpose and methods used in training.
2. Introduce new patients.	Put new patients at ease by asking whether they would prefer being called by their first or last names.
3. Solicit orientation from experienced patients who can explain social skills training to new patients.	Fill in any gaps, if necessary, and select patients to give orientation who are clear, coherent, and upbeat.
4. Reward patients for their contributions to the orientation.	Use praise liberally while looking and smiling at patients.
5. Check homework assignments.	Get details of actual performance, determine obstacles and impediments to generalization, and record results on progress notes.
6. Help each patient pinpoint an interpersonal problem, goal, and scene for this session.	Help patients operationalize their problems by asking what? with whom? where? and when?
	Watch for problems: face, hands, voice, eyes, loudness, posture.
7. Target scene and interpersonal situation for dry run roleplay.	Help patient select and plan the situation, usually one that recently occurred or that will soon occur; get details for scene from patient.
8. "Set up" the scene.	Enlist others to act as roleplayers with the designated patient, move furniture, get props.
9. Give instructions for the scene.	Collaborate with patient on what should be done, tell roleplaying helpers how to respond, determine the patient's short- and long-term goals from the situation to be rehearsed.
10. Run the scene as a dry run.	Watch patient carefully, looking for deficits and assets in verbal, nonverbal, and paralinguistic elements of the patient's performances; keep the scene brief.
11. Give positive feedback.	Find something to praise, give praise immediately, solicit positive and corrective feedback from other patients, use blackboard or easel to get everyone to participate in giving ratings and feedback.

(continued)

Table 3-5. *Continued*

What to Do	*How to Do It*
12. Assess receiving, processing, sending skills.	Ask the patient these questions: • What did the other person say? • What was the other person feeling? • What were your short-term goals? • What were your long-term goals? • What other alternatives could you use in this situation? • Would one of these alternatives help you reach your goals?
13. Use a model.	Select model for similarity to "real " person in patient's life, be sure patient watches the model performing by annotating the skills being demonstrated.
14. Ensure that patient has assimilated the demonstrated skills.	Ask patient to report on model's performance.
15. Use another model.	Optional, but a good idea if the "real" person in the patient's life might respond unpredictably or with greater resistance than the first model.
16. Give instructions to patient for next rehearsal or rerun.	Concentrate on one or two behaviors that need improvement, ask patient to pinpoint the behaviors that are to be improved.
17. Rerun scene.	Use coaching, including hand signals and whispered prompts and praise as scene unfolds.
18. Give summary positive feedback.	Do it immediately, enlist others to join in praising patient, be specific in praising the improved behavioral elements in the patient's roleplayed performance, use blackboard or easel to point out improvement over earlier performance.
19. Give real-life assignment.	Make out assignment card, give clear instructions, keep it simple, invite patient to anticipate any obstacles in carrying out the assignment.
20. Choose another patient for the training sequence and return to step 1.	Ask for a volunteer first, select someone if no one volunteers.

brochure for your use in familiarizing new patients with social skills training and creating favorable expectations.

As we open a typical social skills training session, we will continue our clinical encounters with the patients we met in Chapter 2—Mark, Karen, Ted, Carol, and Allen. Nancy Jones, a clinical psychologist, is the therapist. The group has just assembled to begin one of its twice-weekly meetings. Mark, a newly recruited member, sits on one of the chairs, slightly apart from the rest of the patients and looks just a bit apprehensive.

Therapist: Good morning, all. Let's get our meeting underway. Before we see how well everyone did on their assignments from last time, I'd like to introduce Mark, a new patient for our group. Karen, would you please tell Mark about what we do here in social skills training?

(Karen has been coming to these social skills training sessions for four weeks. She is reticent with the therapist and other group members and complains about being anxious about doing even simple kinds of activities, for example, beginning conversations with others, asking for assistance from others. Before starting social skills training, she was fast becoming a recluse.)

Karen: (Pauses, looks down at her hands for a moment before answering) Well, we, ah, we kind of learn to talk to others better and solve problems we're having with other people. We learn to use our hands (gestures with one hand), make good eye contact (glances up at Mark and the therapist), and speak louder. And we do homework.

Therapist: Great, Karen! Ted, would you add to what Karen said?

(Ted has only been in the group for a week. He often gets angry and upset with other people. He decided to seek social skills training because he recently lost his third roommate in six months and has begun to realize that he alienates other people, including his co-workers. His boss has told him to improve his relations with workmates or else risk being fired.)

Ted: I don't know. Karen described it.

Therapist: Well, can you think of some of the other things we focus on?

Ted: You mean like solving our problems by looking at alternatives for communicating? And whether or not we look mad?

Therapist: Right, Ted. We concentrate on facial expression and problem solving, too. When you talk to someone, they get a lot of information from seeing the kind of expression on your face. How loud we talk and our tone of voice are really important, too. Ted, how is voice tone different from voice loudness?

Ted: Why don't you pick on someone else?

Therapist: Because you're doing really well. You've only been here a short time, and you've learned a lot.

Ted: But I'm not the only one here. Loudness is, ah, like when you shout or whisper. What's the other one?

Therapist: Voice tone.

Ted: Yeah. Tone is like when people whine, like Carol does, or if you sound angry, like you say I do a lot. But I'm not.

Therapist: That's exactly right, Ted. Sometimes people get the wrong idea about us because of the way we say things—and they don't hear what we really are trying to say. Thanks, Ted. Carol, would you tell Mark how we do all this?

(Carol has attended six sessions of the social skills training group. Her long-term goal of getting a job has been broken down into smaller steps, with an initial goal being to succeed as an unpaid volunteer at a senior citizen's center. She has practiced going through an interview with the person in charge of recruiting volunteers in the group and was given an assignment to go to the senior center and apply as a volunteer. She has come punctually to the training sessions and has participated actively in her own training as well as in roleplaying scenes for other group members.)

Carol: You mean like how we go into the middle of the room and pretend to do things? And how we pick other people here to be like the people we would really be talking to outside? Is that what you mean? And I don't whine anymore, either!

Therapist: Very good, Carol. The most important thing is that we practice here how to show and tell others what we really feel in a positive way. And Karen mentioned homework. Everyone gets some homework every time we meet. That's so we can try out in real life what we practiced here and see how well it works. Any questions, Mark?

Mark: I don't know. I can't remember all that stuff. Can't I just watch for a while? I'm not sure I want to get up in front of everybody and do things all wrong.

Therapist: That's OK, Mark, we don't expect you to remember all this right now. And we won't ask you to do much this first session—maybe just introduce yourself to someone, and maybe watch others rehearse their situations so you can tell them how well you think they did. Do you think you can handle that?

Mark: Yeah. OK—I guess so. I don't feel so great right now. I'm kind of nervous.

Bob: I understand. Everyone feels a little strange when we start something new like this. But you can watch the rest of us, and you'll see how enjoyable it is.

Carol: It is fun, Mark. If I can do it, anyone can.

Therapist: Carol was nervous like you, Mark, when she joined the Social Skills Group. Now she's finding that the training is paying off for her.

Just to review, notice in the example above how the therapist called on group members to describe the purposes, content, and procedures of the group to the newcomer. When patients contribute to the orientation, the leader always reinforces their efforts with thanks or praise. Finding something to reward after each patient's contribution is very important for the skills trainer to remember. Patients learn to do this with each other both by example and direct instruction. Thus we take advantage of the need to introduce a new person and to review the purpose of the training for everyone. By the time patients have been involved for a few weeks, you will find that they have learned the main concepts of social skills training and, with a little prompting, can put them into words. Having patients give the bulk of the introduction to social skills training has another value. It creates credible and realistic expectations for the new patient, expectations of active participation in the class, giving and receiving feedback on behaviors, and carrying out assignments.

When you introduce a new patient to the group, you should see to it that you explain why we practice behaviors, particularly the nonverbal ones, like eye contact, gestures, postures, voice tone, and loudness. You should also emphasize the importance of conveying our feelings to others, understanding their feelings, developing alternatives for coping with problems, and seeing the necessity for rehearsal and homework assignments.

The next task in the session is to check on the assignments that were given during the previous session. Go around the room, and check on each patient in turn. You will have a record of each assignment on the social skills training records sheet, and it is very easy to go through the sheets one at a time. Alternatively, you can check on each member's previous assignment when that person's time comes for setting a new goal and working on it during behavioral rehearsal. Everyone soon comes to realize that how well you do on the assignments is the best gauge of progress. It should be a time of good humor and lots of positive strokes. Applause and cheers often break out spontaneously, which set the tone for the rest of the session.

As we rejoin the social skills training session, we hear the therapist say:

Therapist: Let's check on assignments before we go any further. Carol, you were going to find out about becoming a volunteer at the senior citizen's center. You were going to take the bus there and get an interview. How did it go?

Carol: I did pretty bad. I got on the wrong bus and the driver was mean. When I found the right bus and got to the senior citizen's center, the lady who picks the volunteer workers was gone. (Her voice breaks and she whines.) And then I had to get the bus again, but I didn't have the right change. The bus driver wouldn't let me on, so I had to go into a store to get change and then had to wait for the next bus. I got home real late, and my mother was mad. I want to do something constructive with my free time, but I can't do it. I can't do all this. It's not worth all the headaches and hassles.

Therapist: Carol, I think you did very well. You had a tough time. We've all had problems with impolite bus drivers, haven't we? (Mark and Ted agree vigorously.) I'd like to know more about what happened with this bus driver. What did he do to make you so upset?

Notice how the therapist interrupted Carol as she began to catastrophize and move away from an objective report of her assignment followed by problem solving. First, she complimented Carol on doing a good job. Assignments in the real world can go wrong, but most times, if the leaders have brought patients along gradually, with lots of practice and increasingly difficult assignments, the patients will discover that they have hidden reserves and talents they may have either forgotten or never discovered. In this case, Carol needed to see the positive value of her coping efforts. The therapist also probes for details of the incident with the bus driver to pinpoint just what went wrong.

Asking for specifics gives you the details you will need to zero in on how the assignment was carried out and what additional know-how and skills the patient requires for improved functioning. Carol needs to get her facts straight about the buses she will take, to have the right fare ready, and most important, to remain calm, yet assertive, in the face of an angry authority figure—even a city bus driver. She has learned some skills, but there is still more to be done.

Carol: I thought it was the number 21 bus that I was supposed to get on, and I wanted to make sure, you know, to ask the driver. But I didn't have the right change in my hand, and he kept saying "C'mon lady, you're holding everybody up" and looking angry. So I just went and sat down. I was embarrassed in front of all those people, and I dropped my money on the floor. I should have been on the 31 bus.

Ted: I don't let them push me around. I give it right back! I get p.o.-ed when they pull that crap. I got thrown off the bus once.

Therapist: Yes, Ted you're right. It does make you mad when bus drivers aren't helpful or when they get nasty. We might just use that as a practice scene for Carol. Would you be willing to roleplay the part of the bus driver?

Notice how the therapist finds something to praise, even in Ted's outburst. She acknowledges Ted's anger and asks him to help in a practice scene with Carol.

Therapist: What's that paper in your hand, Carol? Is it something you can share with the group?

Carol: Oh. It's an application to be a volunteer at the senior citizen's center. I remembered that you wanted me to bring something back to show that I went there. So I got an application form.

Therapist: Carol, that's just great! You did a great job! You didn't get discouraged when you had trouble on the bus. You got to your destination, and you brought back an application. I think you did beautifully. You deserve a hand. (The therapist applauds, followed by group members. Carol, confused, reacts shyly but then smiles.) What would you like to practice today?

Carol: Oh, I guess how to talk to bus drivers and not cry. I got all flustered and began crying, or maybe I could practice once more the interview for being a volunteer. I didn't get the interview last week.

Therapist: OK, Carol. (She makes a note on Carol's Progress Note.) Let's do the bus driver thing. If we have time we can go over the interview. My record sheet here says that you did very nicely on the interview the last time you practiced it here.

Therapist: Ted, you were going to start conversations with at least two people at your board-and-care home and give at least one compliment to the people while you were talking to them. And you were going to get them to sign your assignment card. Do you have your card, Ted?

Ted: I did it. (Searches through his pockets, pulls a folded, battered 3″×5″ card out of his jeans and hands it to Nancy.) But I only got one initial. I forgot to get the other one. But I did both of them. I felt kind of dumb asking people for their signature or initials or whatever. Freaky.

Therapist: Sounds like you did pretty well, Ted, even if it is a little awkward to ask people to sign your card. Tell us about the conversations.

Ted: Well, I talked to Mr. Bradley, the guy who runs the house I'm staying in. I told him I like the way he lets us decorate our rooms and stuff. A lot of people won't let you put up posters of rock groups. He acted real surprised. Especially when I had him sign my card. Then I talked to the new guy here, what's his name?

Mark: Mark.

Ted: Yeah, Mark. He lives at my board-and-care home. I asked him where he went to school. And stuff like that.

Therapist: Were you able to give at least one compliment to Mark?

Ted: Yeah. I told him I liked the shirt he had on the other day.

Therapist: Mark, Ted didn't have you sign his assignment card. Did he talk to you?

Ted: I talked to him. You don't believe me?

Mark: Yes, he did. I remember him asking me about the shirt.

Therapist: Sounds like you completed your homework. What would you like to work on in this session?

Ted: I'll show you how to deal with bus drivers, how about that?

Therapist: You can help when we work on that problem with Carol, but what problem situations would you like to work on for yourself?

Ted: I don't know. I did OK on the compliments thing.

Therapist: That's true, Ted. You know, something that's related is learning how to give constructive criticism—how to tell someone you want them to change what they do because it annoys or offends you— without getting angry or getting the other person angry or hurt.

Ted: OK. Whatever.

(As you can see, Ted is a real handful. He apparently completed his assignment, and he was pretty specific about the details of his talks with Mr. Bradley and Mark. He doesn't volunteer any situations he wants to work on, but the therapist is ready with a generic communication skill that is part of Ted's long-term goal—positive, effective communication, without the fireworks.)

Therapist: (Checking her own clipboard) Karen, your homework assignment was to go to the store, buy four items, and ask the store manager if he could stock a particular kind of cereal that you like. Were you able to do that?

Karen: (Looks down at her hands) I got the four things. But the person in front of me in the checkout counter was slow, and I was stuck in that little space and I got real anxious so I just paid and left. Here's the cash register receipt.

Therapist: (Taking receipt) Very good, Karen. You stayed long enough to complete a purchase even though you felt anxious. Would you like to practice making that request of the manager again?

Karen: Sure. I think I can do it if I don't get trapped again. I don't like standing in that narrow space they have around the checkout counter. I want to scream.

Therapist: Well, we can set it up so that it can be pretty realistic so you can practice and stay calm at the same time and get the most out of this session. All right. Who's next? Allen? (Consulting his clipboard) What was your assignment?

(Allen has been coming to these sessions for seven weeks. He is less withdrawn, and his engagement in the training has been accompanied by a dramatic decrease in his mannerisms and self-talk. He still speaks so softly and indistinctly that it is difficult to converse with him.)

Allen: (Doesn't respond. He closes his eyes and it is difficult to tell whether he is trying to formulate an answer or if he is avoiding the question. The therapist walks over and stands next to him. She bends over, looks at Allen's face and speaks directly, but not loudly, to engage his attention.)

Therapist: Allen, can you recall what your assignment was for last session?

Allen: (Very softly) Cookout.

Therapist: Cookout?

Allen: (Opens his eyes but looks out the window.) Yeah, to talk to my sister about the family reunion and cookout.

Therapist: Right! That's what I have down here. Your whole family was having a big get-together and cookout, and you were going to ask your sister if you could help prepare for it. What were you supposed to do when you talked to her about the cookout?

Allen: (His voice becomes more audible.) Talk louder . . . and stay on the subject. I was supposed to tell her that I wanted to help out.

Therapist: Do you have your card? Let me check your assignment card.

Allen: (Fishes in his pockets, checks them all, and finally pulls out a crumpled card. He hands it to the therapist.)

Therapist: (Reads card) This is very good, Allen. Your sister reports that you spoke to her for at least two minutes about helping with the cookout. She also says that she could hear you most of the time and that you stayed on the subject, or on target, as we say. I'm very pleased. And your sister gives very clear reports!

Allen: She said I could help make the potato salad.

Therapist: I'm glad you carried through on the homework. I know that it took a lot of effort, Allen, but it paid off because you reached your goal of helping with the family picnic. Did you succeed in obtaining your longer-term goal? Do you have anything in mind that you would like to work on today?

Allen: You mean to reduce the tension in the family by participating more?

Therapist: That's right, and also gradually to take small steps toward greater independence. Knowing how to prepare food is important for anyone who eventually wants to live on his own.

Allen: Yeah. I guess I took a step toward my long-term goal too.

Therapist: Great! Allen, do you want to choose another goal for today's session that deals with your family situation or perhaps go back on working on your basic conversation skills again?

Allen: (Looks down and mumbles an inaudible response.)

Therapist: (Leaning toward Allen) I couldn't hear you Allen.

Allen: I don't care.

Therapist: Perhaps we'd better work on some of your conversation skills again this time. Let's see what we've done before. OK, from the record here, it looks like Allen could use some more practice with voice loudness and eye contact. And, of course, staying with the subject of the conversation—staying "on target."

THE "DRY RUN" BEHAVIORAL REHEARSAL

At this point in the session, the new patients have been introduced, the purpose of training has been explained to them—and reviewed for everyone else in the social skills group. Most important, the leader has gotten detailed reports from the patients on the homework assignments from the previous session and recorded whether or not they were accomplished. Checking on the homework also helped the patients and therapist to plan the goals and situations to be used in the next training steps. The next task is to engage the patient in active rehearsal of the problematic social situation.

In the subsequent training, we will have each patient go through the following steps in practicing their skills for dealing with the chosen interpersonal situation:

* *Rehearse situation in dry run.* The patient is assisted in setting up a scenario involving the interpersonal target and is encouraged to practice the situation.
* *Provide positive feedback.* The therapist calls on the group to tell the patient what he or she did well in the dry run.
* *Emphasize training in social perception and problem solving.* The patient's receiving, processing, and sending skills are checked and corrected, if necessary.
* *Engage in modeling.* Another patient or a staff person is used to demonstrate another, possibly more effective, way of handling the same scene.
* *Rerun the scene.* The patient goes through the same scene, with specific instructions and coaching for making improvements. Two or three "takes" are typical.
* *Give an assignment.*

First we'll start on a step in the training process that combines assessment with initial efforts at skill building—the "dry run," or initial behavioral rehearsal. In this rehearsal, the patient is asked to enact a scene involving another person with minimal coaching or discussion, which gives the therapist an opportunity to assess the deficits as well as assets of the patient in the simulated encounter. The practice helps the patient overcome anxiety and to practice skills, while at the same time gives the therapist a reasonably accurate picture of the patient's skill level. See Table 3-6 for the specific steps in this phase of social skills training.

Therapist: Carol, you had quite a bit of trouble getting to the senior citizen's center on your last assignment. Will you show us what happened when you got uptight on the bus? We can play it out here and help you make some improvements in coping with rude bus drivers. Who could help us play the part of the bus driver?

Carol: Well, Ted could. He even looks like the driver a little bit.

Therapist: OK, Ted, please come over here and sit in this chair and help Carol by taking the part of the bus driver. (Points to a chair in center of the group and sets up a couple of empty chairs behind it to simulate a bus.) Carol, you pretend you are just getting on the bus.

Carol has picked Ted to play the bus driver because he resembles the bus driver. It's important to have the patient pick someone who matches the real-life person as closely as possible. Age, sex, physical characteristics, and style of communication are important attributes to match for the person who will take the part of the "target" person—the key "other person" in the scene to whom the patient will direct his or her communications. Now the therapist asks Carol to add as many details as possible so that Ted, as bus driver, can play his role realistically.

Therapist: Tell us as much as you can about the first bus driver, the one on the wrong bus. Tell us what you both said and did.

Carol: Well, I was watching the kids in the schoolyard across the street from the bus stop, so I guess I wasn't paying attention. All of a sudden the bus was there, and I couldn't remember if the number was right. I felt confused and got upset. I started to ask the driver if I was on the right bus to the senior citizen's center, but I couldn't remember the cross streets and he was getting mad. So I got on and sat down. I didn't want to bother him while he was driving. They have that sign about not talking to the driver, and I thought I could get him in trouble. I was getting more and more nervous because I didn't see any buildings or landmarks that I recognize. Finally, a lady must have seen how upset I was, and she asked if she could help. She gave me directions on what to do.

Therapist: What did the driver say to you?

Carol: He said "Are you getting on?" And then I said, "Do you go to senior citizen's center?" And he asked where it was, but I couldn't tell him the streets. There were other people behind me trying to get on, and I felt like I was holding them up.

Therapist: OK. Let's do a "dry run" rehearsal of that situation where you're getting on the bus. Ted, you've got a good picture of the job you have as the bus driver, don't you?

Ted: Yup. I've got to keep the bus moving on schedule and can't keep passengers waiting. I'll try to act as businesslike as possible.

Therapist: Fine. Let's run the scene, and we'll see how you do, Carol. Then we'll come up with some ideas for helping you become more effective and less flustered in this type of situation. I want a few of the other group members to stand behind Carol as if you're impatiently waiting to get on the bus. Let it roll anytime you're ready, Carol.

This first runthrough, or "dry run," will show more about how Carol performed than her verbal, retrospective description. In fact, the "dry run" is an excellent assessment tool for observing the patient's social skills and deficits in the situation being roleplayed. All the therapist's clinical sensitivity must be used while observing the behavioral rehearsal unfold—eyes, ears, intuition, and even the proverbial "third ear."

(Carol approaches Ted from the side. Ted is looking forward, out of his "windshield." Carol stands just short of the bus "door" and stops, looking in her purse. Two other patients stand behind her. The therapist stands behind Ted, who is roleplaying the bus driver, to have an unobstructed view of Carol as she goes through the scene.)

Ted: Are you getting on?

Carol: Do you . . . uh . . . go to . . . uh . . .

Ted: What?

Carol: Do you go past the senior citizen's center?

Ted: I don't know. Where is it?

Carol: I . . . uh . . . have a piece of paper somewhere . . .

Mark: (From behind her) Hey lady, I wanna get on. Let's go.

Ted: Would you step to one side? Let some of these others on? (The others go past, pretending to give the driver their fares.) Can you find the address? I have to stay on schedule.

Carol: (Her face flushes noticeably. She starts to respond.) No . . . it's where they take volunteers. I have an appointment.

Ted: I'm sorry, but I really have to get moving. (Carol looks at the therapist as if asking for help. She is breathing rapidly and looks genuinely confused.)

Therapist: Let's cut the action right here.

Table 3-6. Step-by-Step Map for Guiding Therapists Through a Typical Session of Social Skills Training. Boxed steps are for the dry run or initial behavioral rehearsal phase of training.

What to Do	How to Do It
1. Give introduction to social skills training.	Welcome patients, introduce yourself, give a brief description of the purpose and methods used in training.
2. Introduce new patients.	Put new patients at ease by asking whether they would prefer being called by their first or last names.
3. Solicit orientation from experienced patients who can explain social skills training to new patients.	Fill in any gaps, if necessary, and select patients to give orientation who are clear, coherent, and upbeat.
4. Reward patients for their contributions to the orientation.	Use praise liberally while looking and smiling at patients.
5. Check homework assignments.	Get details of actual performance, determine obstacles and impediments to generalization, and record results on progress notes.
6. Help each patient pinpoint an interpersonal problem, goal, and scene for this session.	Help patients operationalize their problems by asking what? with whom? where? and when? Watch for problems: face, hands, voice, eyes, loudness, posture.
7. **Target scene and interpersonal situation for dry run roleplay.**	**Help patient select and plan the situation, usually one that recently occurred or that will soon occur; get details for scene from patient.**
8. **"Set up" the scene.**	**Enlist others to act as roleplayers with the designated patient, move furniture, get props.**
9. **Give instructions for the scene.**	**Collaborate with patient on what should be done, tell roleplaying helpers how to respond, determine the patient's short- and long-term goals from the situation to be rehearsed.**
10. **Run the scene as a dry run.**	**Watch patient carefully, looking for deficits and assets in verbal, nonverbal, and paralinguistic elements of the patient's performances; keep the scene brief.**
11. **Give positive feedback.**	**Find something to praise, give praise immediately, solicit positive and corrective feedback from other patients, use blackboard or easel to get everyone to participate in giving ratings and feedback.**

(continued)

Table 3-6. *Continued*

What to Do	*How to Do It*
12. Assess receiving, processing, sending skills.	Ask the patient these questions: • What did the other person say? • What was the other person feeling? • What were your short-term goals? • What were your long-term goals? • What other alternatives could you use in this situation? • Would one of these alternatives help you reach your goals?
13. Use a model.	Select model for similarity to "real" person in patient's life, be sure patient watches the model performing by annotating the skills being demonstrated.
14. Ensure that patient has assimilated the demonstrated skills.	Ask patient to report on model's performance.
15. Use another model.	Optional, but a good idea if the "real" person in the patient's life might respond unpredictably or with greater resistance than the first model.
16. Give instructions to patient for next rehearsal or rerun.	Concentrate on one or two behaviors that need improvement, ask patient to pinpoint the behaviors that are to be improved.
17. Rerun scene.	Use coaching, including hand signals and whispered prompts and praise as scene unfolds.
18. Give summary positive feedback.	Do it immediately, enlist others to join in praising patient, be specific in praising the improved behavioral elements in the patient's roleplayed performance, use blackboard or easel to point out improvement over earlier performance.
19. Give real-life assignment.	Make out assignment card, give clear instructions, keep it simple, invite patient to anticipate any obstacles in carrying out the assignment.
20. Choose another patient for the training sequence and return to step 1.	Ask for a volunteer first, select someone if no one volunteers.

Carol, as you were playing this scene here, did you feel it was like it was on the bus?

Carol: Yes, it was pretty real. I felt like I was going to cry again, and Ted was pretty much like the driver. I guess I just get flustered around strangers, you know, in front of all those people you don't know.

Therapist: All right. We should stop here and give Carol some positive feedback.

Notice that Nancy, the therapist, cuts off the scene fairly quickly. Scenes contain so much raw information that it's best not to let them go on any longer than is absolutely necessary to draw some conclusions about the performance. If the scene is allowed to continue too long, the focus for the training gets lost in myriad details and irrelevancies. Furthermore, by letting a patient flounder in an awkward effort to recapitulate the problem situation, you are risking that ineffective responses will be perpetuated and that the distress experienced by the patient will interfere with a desire to continue participating in the subsequent training steps.

Here the therapist sees almost at once from Ted's roleplaying that the driver probably isn't any worse than most; he certainly didn't get angry or abusive. Carol, in her frustration and discomfort, most likely misread the bus driver's emotional state. Her "receiving," "processing," and "sending" skills need work. The therapist also knows now that Carol just wasn't prepared for this outing, that she wasn't paying attention to the buses coming and going, that she forgot the number of the bus she was supposed to board, and that she either didn't have the address of her destination or she had misplaced it. Strictly speaking, none of these are social skills, but if Carol better organized her trip before she left home, she wouldn't have become so anxious and confused on the bus.

Carol obviously needs some specific education on how to get around town on public transportation—a fact that the therapist writes down for future planning. The therapist also sees that part of the problem is Carol's deficiencies in dealing with others in public, trying to get her own needs met with others looking on and being impatient. Remaining calm in spite of this pressure is another important element in performing well socially.

GIVING POSITIVE FEEDBACK

Because psychiatric patients often lack intrinsic motivation to learn social skills, positive feedback from the therapist and other group members serves as a key source of motivation. Praise must be administered in liberal doses throughout the training process to compensate for patients' anhedonia and lack of enthusiasm. The therapist utilizes every opportunity to give realistic praise to each patient, including the crucial point immediately after the dry run.

Therapist: (To the group) What did Carol do *well* in this scene? What things did she do *right* here?

Karen: She didn't get mad or cry.

Ted: She looked at the driver when she spoke to him. But she blew it.

Therapist: (Purposely ignoring Ted's critical comment) Yes, she didn't get angry or break down crying, and she kept eye contact with the driver. She also asked the driver clearly if his bus went to the senior citizen's center. Very good, Carol. Now let's size up how you responded to the bus driver.

TRAINING SOCIAL PERCEPTION AND PROBLEM SOLVING

The therapist now has Carol step back from the situation so that she can look at her receiving skills, her goals, and her options. We seldom do this methodically in our busy lives, but social skills training allows us the luxury of time to assess our patients' accuracy or distortions in social perception, their strategies used for reaching their goals, and their ability to generate alternatives for solving social problems. See Table 3-7 for this step in training.

Therapist: Carol, in the dry run we just did, how did you think Ted—taking the bus driver's role—was feeling toward you?

Carol: He looked really annoyed at me, I could tell. He said something like, "If you don't know where it is, I can't help you. I have to get moving."

Therapist: Can you remember what it was that he said *precisely*? Did he yell or scowl at you? What made you think he was angry?

Carol: Uh . . . well . . . actually he said: "I'm sorry, I can't help you if you don't know where you're going."

Therapist: Carol, what do you think the driver was feeling at that moment? Do you still think he was angry?

Carol: Well, no, not exactly. He seemed kind of mean, though. I guess he was more in a rush. I felt foolish.

Ted: That's right, Carol. I was just being businesslike and polite. I did

Table 3-7. Step-by-Step Map for Guiding Therapists Through a Typical Session of Social Skills Training. The boxed step is for the assessment and training of social perception (receiving) and problem solving (processing).

What to Do	How to Do It
1. Give introduction to social skills training.	Welcome patients, introduce yourself, give a brief description of the purpose and methods used in training.
2. Introduce new patients.	Put new patients at ease by asking whether they would prefer being called by their first or last names.
3. Solicit orientation from experienced patients who can explain social skills training to new patients.	Fill in any gaps, if necessary, and select patients to give orientation who are clear, coherent, and upbeat.
4. Reward patients for their contributions to the orientation.	Use praise liberally while looking and smiling at patients.
5. Check homework assignments.	Get details of actual performance, determine obstacles and impediments to generalization, and record results on progress notes.
6. Help each patient pinpoint an interpersonal problem, goal, and scene for this session.	Help patients operationalize their problems by asking what? with whom? where? and when? Watch for problems: face, hands, voice, eyes, loudness, posture.
7. Target scene and interpersonal situation for dry run roleplay.	Help patient select and plan the situation, usually one that recently occurred or that will soon occur; get details for scene from patient.
8. "Set up" the scene.	Enlist others to act as roleplayers with the designated patient, move furniture, get props.
9. Give instructions for the scene.	Collaborate with patient on what should be done, tell roleplaying helpers how to respond, determine the patient's short- and long-term goals from the situation to be rehearsed.
10. Run the scene as a dry run.	Watch patient carefully, looking for deficits and assets in verbal, nonverbal, and paralinguistic elements of the patient's performances; keep the scene brief.
11. Give positive feedback.	Find something to praise, give praise immediately, solicit positive and corrective feedback from other patients, use blackboard or easel to get everyone to participate in giving ratings and feedback.

(continued)

Table 3-7. *Continued*

What to Do	*How to Do It*
12. Assess receiving, processing, sending skills.	**Ask the patient these questions:** • **What did the other person say?** • **What was the other person feeling?** • **What were your short-term goals?** • **What were your long-term goals?** • **What other alternatives could you use in this situation?** • **Would one of these alternatives help you reach your goals?**

13. Use a model.	Select model for similarity to "real" person in patient's life, be sure patient watches the model performing by annotating the skills being demonstrated.
14. Ensure that patient has assimilated the demonstrated skills.	Ask patient to report on model's performance.
15. Use another model.	Optional, but a good idea if the "real" person in the patient's life might respond unpredictably or with greater resistance than the first model.
16. Give instructions to patient for next rehearsal or rerun.	Concentrate on one or two behaviors that need improvement, ask patient to pinpoint the behaviors that are to be improved.
17. Rerun scene.	Use coaching, including hand signals and whispered prompts and praise as scene unfolds.
18. Give summary positive feedback.	Do it immediately, enlist others to join in praising patient, be specific in praising the improved behavioral elements in the patient's roleplayed performance, use blackboard or easel to point out improvement over earlier performance.
19. Give real-life assignment.	Make out assignment card, give clear instructions, keep it simple, invite patient to anticipate any obstacles in carrying out the assignment.
20. Choose another patient for the training sequence and return to step 1.	Ask for a volunteer first, select someone if no one volunteers.

have to keep the bus on schedule, but I was trying to help you. You got so upset. You weren't even aware of my helpfulness.

Therapist: It's all right to be afraid and anxious when you're not sure of what you're doing. So it's possible that the bus driver was rushed and wanted to stay on schedule. You know, bus drivers get in trouble if they don't stay on schedule. Did he raise his voice at you?

Carol: No. I guess that I must have been so upset that I lost track of what was really happening. I thought he was mad because I felt foolish and scared.

The therapist helps Carol understand that in getting flustered and confused, she projected her worries and fears onto the bus driver who probably wasn't as rude as she had indicated at first. Some significant facts come out when the therapist helps Carol to focus more specifically on the actual interactions. The clarifying nature of the therapist's questions helps Carol to learn to tune in better to others' emotions.

Therapist: Carol, now that we've clarified how the bus driver was feeling, let's see if we can help you come up with an alternative and more effective way of dealing with this situation. What do you think your short-term goal was in this situation?

Carol: I just wanted to get to where I was going, to the senior center.

Therapist: Yes, but you also needed some help. You lost the address!

Carol: I guess so. I have to get the driver to help me out, if he can.

Therapist: So, for this situation, getting some help from a busy bus driver is your short-term goal. What could you do differently to reach your short-term goal?

Carol: Be better prepared and not get so anxious when things go wrong. I get so mad at myself, but I don't seem to be able to prevent myself from getting uptight and choked.

Therapist: Being better prepared for a bus trip is one good alternative. But even if you've choked up, you might still be able to communicate your need to the bus driver. Let's ask Ted if he has any ideas.

Ted: I felt pretty rushed. There were all these people trying to get on, and I knew I had to make my schedule, and here was Carol, and she didn't seem to know where she was going and she was in the way. I think a real bus driver, even a really nice one, would have trouble with someone like Carol. She's got to shape up.

Therapist: (Sidestepping the critical tone in Ted's response) Ted, how might Carol shape up and be more effective, despite being anxious in that situation. How would you be receptive to a passenger with a problem like Carol's? What could she say?

Ted: Well, she could give the bus driver some more information about the senior center and ask him politely to assist her in locating it.

Therapist: Excellent suggestion, Ted. Carol, do you think that kind of approach would help you meet your short-term goal, even if you weren't prepared with the directions? (Carol nods an assent.) And how about your long-term goal?

Carol: I don't know . . . you mean to get to know how to use the buses?

Therapist: Yes, and become more independent. That is your long-term goal. It will give you a sense of confidence that you haven't had. What other skills can you learn to help you reach your short- and long-term goals?

Carol: Lots of practice? I think I need more help with doing this.

Therapist: Yes, that certainly will help. Let's also review some of the ways to be personally effective with others. Look at the list of skills on the blackboard, and I'll get some feedback for you from others in the group.

(The therapist now refers to a list of the verbal and nonverbal elements of communicating effectively. On a blackboard there is a list as shown in Figure 3-3.)

Therapist: What could Carol have done to improve in that situation?

Ted: Everything.

Therapist: Now you know we have to be a lot more specific if we can help her improve. Let's begin by rating Carol's performance on the behaviors we have on the board here. Karen, why would you rate Carol's eye contact as needing improvement?

Karen: Well, she was looking around, she was looking in her purse, and when she got upset, she looked away.

Therapist: What could she do to improve? So she needs improvement?

Karen: Well, if she had her money and her address ready, maybe she wouldn't have to look in her purse.

Therapist: Good feedback, Karen. Let's go on. How about Carol's hand gestures? Ted, why do you feel that Carol could improve her gestures as she communicates?

Ted: Because she was messing around in her purse, and she couldn't use her hands.

Therapist: That's true, Ted. Good observation. What could she have done differently?

Ted: She could have shrugged her shoulders and put her palms up when asking the driver for assistance.

The therapist acknowledges Ted's constructive suggestion and goes on through the rest of the items on the wall poster, quickly getting evaluative comments and suggestions from all present. When someone rates a behavior as very good or very poor, she asks for specifics and prompts patients to formulate their criticism in a constructive manner. Group feedback also tends to keep the other patients in the group alert and involved in the training process and promotes vicarious learning while they are waiting their turn to rehearse. It motivates them to pay attention and strengthens group cohesion.

USING A MODEL

The therapist is now ready for the next important step—choosing a person who will run through the same scene to show Carol how to incorporate the suggestions and corrective feedback just provided to improve the handling of the same situation. Even though the social skills you will be teaching are relatively simple, any social contact is very complicated. If you had to list all the differences between the way two people ask for the correct time, you would be able to fill pages of subtle distinctions. *The most effective way to teach complex social behavior is through modeling and imitation.* There are probably as many ways to deal with any given situation as there are available people to play the scene, but one or two are generally sufficient.

The important thing to remember is not to skip this step. It is especially crucial for patients with learning disabilities and major deficiencies in needed skills—like persons with schizophrenia and other chronic and serious mental disorders. Everyone gains something from watching a model. See Table 3-8 for the steps to use.

Therapist: Karen, would you mind showing us how you would handle this situation? Pretend that you have just discovered that you have lost your directions just as Carol did. Show us how you would get the information you need. Highlight for Carol good eye contact and some appropriate hand gestures while you tell the bus driver of your dilemma and make a direct appeal for his assistance. (The therapist picked Karen as a model because of her similarity to Carol in age, and, of course, sex. Also Karen's social skills, while better than Carol's, are not so vastly superior as to make her an implausible model. As a peer with problems of her own, she is a good person for Carol to emulate.)

Therapist: Let's do this again. Passengers, get behind Karen. OK. Go!

(The therapist takes Carol by the elbow and maneuvers her around to the left side of Ted, who is still roleplaying the bus driver. She makes sure that Carol is watching Karen during this modeling sequence.)

When you use a model, move your patient around to this vantage point. Be sure you have clearly told the patient what you want her (or him) to observe before the model begins, and ask for this information to be repeated back to you. Don't be afraid to whisper in your observing patient's ear during the action to draw attention to particularly good elements of the model's performance. Asking the patient to report on what he or she saw after the modeling performance further drives home the important points. Sometimes you may find that you have to guide the patient's head or gaze—ever so gently—in the right direction to ensure that he or she is observing the model's performance.

Ted: You getting on, lady?

Karen: (Looks in her purse) Ah . . . yes, at least I think I am. (She turns to the other "passengers" behind her.) Why don't you all go ahead? I'm trying to find my directions. Driver, I seem to have lost my directions. I think I'm supposed to be on this bus, but I'm not sure. I'm trying to find an agency called Senior Citizens' Center. It's a place where old folks socialize, a charitable organization, and I'm going for a job interview. Do you know if I'm on the right bus?

Ted: I dunno, lady. I got to keep my schedule.

Karen: I know, driver. I'm terribly sorry to bother you, but I really need some help to get there. I might miss out on a job.

Ted: Well, uh, do you know what street it's on?

Karen: No, that was on my directions. I saw it, but I didn't memorize it.

Ted: Well, shoot, lady! That makes it tough. You ever been there before? You know what it looks like even?

Karen: Yes, I was there once, last week. All I can remember is that it has this big blue awning in front.

Ted: Hey, I've seen that place. But you're on the wrong bus. Take the 21 bus to Jackson. That place is about a half a block down on your right when you get off. The number 21 bus will be here in about ten minutes. Now I really have to get going.

Karen: The 21 to Jackson. Thank you for being so patient.

Therapist: (The therapist signals "cut" and brings Carol around to the center of the group again.) Thank you, Karen. Carol, what were the things that Karen did that made that scene go better?

Carol: Oh, she did better than I did. She didn't get upset. She kept looking at the driver and her voice tone was better than mine. I was going to cry, and I couldn't talk right. And she let the people on and then got him to give directions.

Therapist: Yes, that's a lot. Very good. I'm glad you were able to pick up on all that. Karen also expressed her concern with hand gestures—did

Table 3-8. Step-by-Step Map for Guiding Therapists Through a Typical Session of Social Skills Training. Boxed steps are for the modeling phase of training.

What to Do	How to Do It
1. Give introduction to social skills training.	Welcome patients, introduce yourself, give a brief description of the purpose and methods used in training.
2. Introduce new patients.	Put new patients at ease by asking whether they would prefer being called by their first or last names.
3. Solicit orientation from experienced patients who can explain social skills training to new patients.	Fill in any gaps, if necessary, and select patients to give orientation who are clear, coherent, and upbeat.
4. Reward patients for their contributions to the orientation.	Use praise liberally while looking and smiling at patients.
5. Check homework assignments.	Get details of actual performance, determine obstacles and impediments to generalization, and record results on progress notes.
6. Help each patient pinpoint an interpersonal problem, goal, and scene for this session.	Help patients operationalize their problems by asking what? with whom? where? and when?
	Watch for problems: face, hands, voice, eyes, loudness, posture.
7. Target scene and interpersonal situation for dry run roleplay.	Help patient select and plan the situation, usually one that recently occurred or that will soon occur; get details for scene from patient.
8. "Set up" the scene.	Enlist others to act as roleplayers with the designated patient, move furniture, get props.
9. Give instructions for the scene.	Collaborate with patient on what should be done, tell roleplaying helpers how to respond, determine the patient's short- and long-term goals from the situation to be rehearsed.
10. Run the scene as a dry run.	Watch patient carefully, looking for deficits and assets in verbal, nonverbal, and paralinguistic elements of the patient's performances; keep the scene brief.
11. Give positive feedback.	Find something to praise, give praise immediately, solicit positive and corrective feedback from other patients, use blackboard or easel to get everyone to participate in giving ratings and feedback.

(continued)

Table 3-8. *Continued*

What to Do	*How to Do It*
12. Assess receiving, processing, sending skills.	Ask the patient these questions: • What did the other person say? • What was the other person feeling? • What were your short-term goals? • What were your long-term goals? • What other alternatives could you use in this situation? • Would one of these alternatives help you reach your goals?
13. Use a model.	**Select model for similarity to "real" person in patient's life, be sure patient watches the model performing by annotating the skills being demonstrated.**
14. Ensure that patient has assimilated the demonstrated skills.	**Ask patient to report on model's performance.**
15. Use another model.	**Optional, but a good idea if the "real" person in the patient's life might respond unpredictably or with greater resistance than the first model.**
16. Give instructions to patient for next rehearsal or rerun.	Concentrate on one or two behaviors that need improvement, ask patient to pinpoint the behaviors that are to be improved.
17. Rerun scene.	Use coaching, including hand signals and whispered prompts and praise as scene unfolds.
18. Give summary positive feedback.	Do it immediately, enlist others to join in praising patient, be specific in praising the improved behavioral elements in the patient's roleplayed performance, use blackboard or easel to point out improvement over earlier performance.
19. Give real-life assignment.	Make out assignment card, give clear instructions, keep it simple, invite patient to anticipate any obstacles in carrying out the assignment.
20. Choose another patient for the training sequence and return to step 1.	Ask for a volunteer first, select someone if no one volunteers.

you see that? Now I want you to try the scene again, but this time I want you to remain as relaxed as you can. Making eye contact with the driver will reduce your nervousness. Don't fumble with your purse. Be sure to use a few hand gestures. I'm going to stand behind the bus driver while you explain your problem and appeal to him for help. Remember, as a passenger you have the right to ask for directions of a bus driver, and he has a responsibility to be helpful to customers.
Carol: I guess so.

The therapist directed this runthrough with Karen as the model for Carol to imitate. She made sure that Carol was paying attention to Karen by moving her around the target person in the scene and whispering pointers to her as Carol demonstrated the desired skills. As soon as the scene was over, the therapist again called on Carol to check whether Carol had observed and assimilated the nonverbal behaviors as well as the content of Karen's speech.

RERUN BEHAVIORAL REHEARSAL WITH COACHING

To finish this skills training sequence with Carol, the therapist will ask Carol to practice the same scene again to determine if Carol has assimilated the improvement shown by the model. If she hasn't, she'll need some prompting and instructions. For patients with long-standing and serious mental disorders, direct their attention to just one of the elements of social skills to be learned—eye contact or voice tone, for instance. Limiting the focus of learning is particularly important for patients with conceptual disorganization or thought disorder. You can feel more confident in having a higher-functioning patient try to work on three or more skills at once in a scene. If you make a mistake and try to go too far too fast, you will see the results in confusion and frustration. It's better to go more slowly; in fact, you will often see several aspects of the performance improve, even if you have given instructions to work on just one or two. See the steps in Table 3-9 to guide you through the rerun.

There are a few hand signals that we find useful in coaching patients to improve their skill level. Remember, you must be standing where you can easily see the patient's face, and use clearly agreed-upon sign language to give instructions during the scene. This speeds up the training enormously, since you don't have to interrupt the action to give more

Table 3-9. Step-by-Step Map for Guiding Therapists Through a Typical Session of Social Skills Training Session. The boxed steps cover the repeat behavioral rehearsal, or "rerun," that required active coaching by the therapist.

What to Do	How to Do It
1. Give introduction to social skills training.	Welcome patients, introduce yourself, give a brief description of the purpose and methods used in training.
2. Introduce new patients.	Put new patients at ease by asking whether they would prefer being called by their first or last names.
3. Solicit orientation from experienced patients who can explain social skills training to new patients.	Fill in any gaps, if necessary, and select patients to give orientation who are clear, coherent, and upbeat.
4. Reward patients for their contributions to the orientation.	Use praise liberally while looking and smiling at patients.
5. Check homework assignments.	Get details of actual performance, determine obstacles and impediments to generalization, and record results on progress notes.
6. Help each patient pinpoint an interpersonal problem, goal, and scene for this session.	Help patients operationalize their problems by asking what? with whom? where? and when? Watch for problems: face, hands, voice, eyes, loudness, posture.
7. Target scene and interpersonal situation for dry run roleplay.	Help patient select and plan the situation, usually one that recently occurred or that will soon occur; get details for scene from patient.
8. "Set up" the scene.	Enlist others to act as roleplayers with the designated patient, move furniture, get props.
9. Give instructions for the scene.	Collaborate with patient on what should be done, tell roleplaying helpers how to respond, determine the patient's short- and long-term goals from the situation to be rehearsed.
10. Run the scene as a dry run.	Watch patient carefully, looking for deficits and assets in verbal, nonverbal, and paralinguistic elements of the patient's performances; keep the scene brief.
11. Give positive feedback.	Find something to praise, give praise immediately, solicit positive and corrective feedback from other patients, use blackboard or easel to get everyone to participate in giving ratings and feedback.

(continued)

Table 3-9. *Continued*

What to Do	How to Do It
12. Assess receiving, processing, sending skills.	Ask the patient these questions: • What did the other person say? • What was the other person feeling? • What were your short-term goals? • What were your long-term goals? • What other alternatives could you use in this situation? • Would one of these alternatives help you reach your goals?
13. Use a model.	Select model for similarity to "real " person in patient's life, be sure patient watches the model performing by annotating the skills being demonstrated.
14. Ensure that patient has assimilated the demonstrated skills.	Ask patient to report on model's performance.
15. Use another model.	Optional, but a good idea if the "real" person in the patient's life might respond unpredictably or with greater resistance than the first model.
16. Give instructions to patient for next rehearsal or rerun.	**Concentrate on one or two behaviors that need improvement, ask patient to pinpoint the behaviors that are to be improved.**
17. Rerun scene.	**Use coaching, including hand signals and whispered prompts and praise as scene unfolds.**
18. Give summary positive feedback.	**Do it immediately, enlist others to join in praising patient, be specific in praising the improved behavioral elements in the patient's roleplayed performance, use blackboard or easel to point out improvement over earlier performance.**
19. Give real-life assignment.	Make out assignment card, give clear instructions, keep it simple, invite patient to anticipate any obstacles in carrying out the assignment.
20. Choose another patient for the training sequence and return to step 1.	Ask for a volunteer first, select someone if no one volunteers.

instructions. Common hand signals used in social skills training are depicted graphically in Figure 3-7.

There are many different ways of giving instructions during the training itself. Technically, this is called prompting, but it comes down to the therapist giving the patient cues. We have used electronic gadgets, such as a remote transmitter and receiver in the patient's ear, but simple hand signals are less confusing and more fun, and they add to the general activity level, helping to keep attention focused on the action. The technique of actually whispering in the patient's ear during the scene is especially helpful when hand signals can't cue content very easily and a patient is almost at a loss for something to say. Hand signals can tell *how* to say something, but not *what* to say.

The other instructional technique used in the rerun behavioral re-

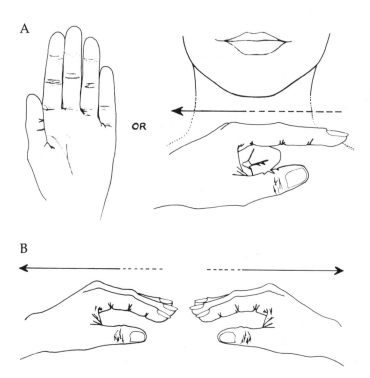

FIGURE 3-7. Hand signals are a convenient and effective means of coaching the patient's improved performance in the "rerun" or repeat behavioral rehearsal of social skills training. The drawings are keyed to the code that follows, indicating the meaning of each signal.
A. Forefinger moving across the throat or palm outstretched at patient = "Stop the action!"
B. Hands moving horizontally as if pulling taffy between them = "Slow down your pace of speaking."

C

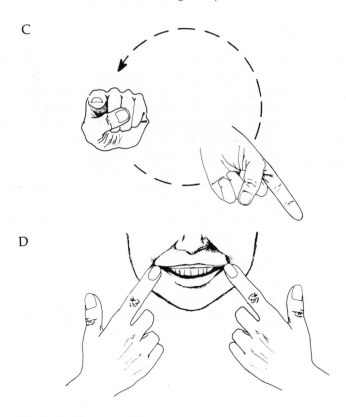

D

Figure 3-7. *Continued*
C. One hand moving fast in a right circle = "Speed up the pace of speaking."
D. Fingers manipulating the mouth in an exaggerated smile or frown = "Smile or look serious."

hearsal is positive "on-line" feedback. Thus, when a patient is making approximations to the desired skills and showing even slight improvements during the rerun, the therapist leans toward the patient and whispers in his or her ear, "Very good" (specifies the behavior), or "Keep up the good voice volume," or "Terrific!" (specifies the behavior). Hand signals can also be used for conveying approval and praise, such as a "V" signal or "thumbs up" signal. If the patient still shows deficits in the rerun, even after modeling, the therapist can use "on-line" prompts to facilitate the acquisition of targeted skills. For example, a therapist can cue the patient by whispering in his ear, "Tell the person what he did and how it made you feel."

Prompting, cues, and praise for the repeat performance are termed "coaching," since they are similar to the actions of athletic or drama coaches. With active and timely coaching during the rerun, it is close to

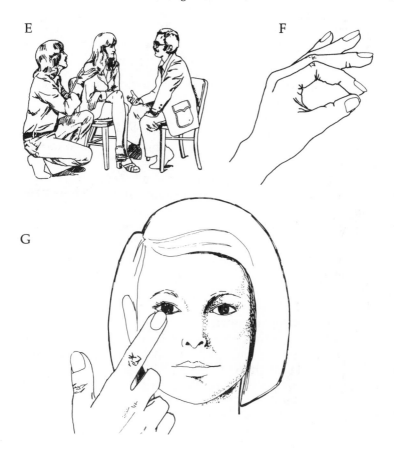

Figure 3-7. *Continued*
E. Both palms up, moving up and down or both palms down, moving down and up = "Talk louder" or "Talk softer."
F. Forefinger and thumb touching, forming a circle, the other fingers extended = "Great job, good work, keep it up."
G. Finger pointed to corner of eye = "Make more eye contact."
Drawings courtesy of Jeff Moersfelder.

impossible for the patient not to improve—at least a little. As an active-directive therapist, you are employing all the known learning techniques to promote some small increment in social competence. Even your close physical proximity to the patient as the scene unfolds gives emotional support and encouragement that aids motivation and morale.

Let's see how, as Nancy has Carol run through the scene once more. In fact she might actually repeat it two or three more times if there is time in the session. More and varied practice is always better! For example, it would be useful to teach Carol how to deal with a variety of bus drivers, from courteous and helpful to surly and rude.

Therapist: We'll do this once more. Carol, take your place. Everyone get set to do it again. Go!

Ted: Lady, are you gettin' on?

Carol: (Looks in her purse, then looks back at the driver.) I'm not sure. I think I've misplaced my directions. I want to go to the senior citizen's center.

Passengers: Hey, can we get on. How's about it, lady?

Carol: (Looks apprehensively at their outburst) Yes. Sure. Why don't you get on, and then I'll ask the driver for some help.

Ted: Where is this place? Don't you know where you're going?

Carol: I'm terribly sorry. (Looks at him, shrugs, and makes a gesture of impatience with herself.) I don't even remember the address. But it's a big volunteer agency and it has a blue awning outside. They sell used things there.

Ted: I dunno, lady. I got a schedule to keep. Just a sec. I've seen that place. But you're on the wrong bus . . .

(The therapist cuts the scene here as Carol has clearly demonstrated improved coping skills. She is now ready for some final positive feedback, which will be orchestrated by the therapist.)

Therapist: Carol, what were you able to accomplish this time that made you more successful?

Carol: I kept my eyes on Ted and tried to tell him that I needed his help to find my way. I also didn't fiddle with my purse this time and let the others go past before I asked the driver to give me some help.

To reinforce the improvements shown by patients in their repeat rehearsals, the therapist solicits positive feedback from as many of the other group members as feasible. The therapist, Nancy, asks each member of the group to tell Carol clearly what they noticed had improved or remained personally effective. Again, the soliciting of positive feedback is done with careful phraseology, such as, "Ted, tell Carol how her more direct way of asking for your help affected your desire to assist her." These careful directions will reduce the chances of destructive criticism being leveled and keeps the therapist in control of the group process.

Praise, linked to the specific elements of skill that have improved, is also given by the therapist. Even more valuable as reinforcement are the positive evaluations and self-statements made by the patient himself or herself. It is important to keep the praise in proportion to the actual performance—excessively effusive praise will lose its credibility. One person from whom positive feedback should always be solicited is the person who took the part of the "target" in the roleplay—in this case, Ted who, as the bus driver, absorbed the full impact of Carol's improved communication skills.

The therapist then runs through the ratings of the nonverbal behaviors, once again using the blackboard. Carol gets much improved notices from the other group members. The therapist leads the group in a brief round of applause; Carol has done very well, and she has worked hard. All that remains is to give her an assignment to carry out before the next session. Finally, Nancy turns to Carol and prompts her to evaluate her own performance.

Therapist: Carol, what were you able to accomplish this time that made you more successful?

Carol: I kept my eyes on Ted and tried to tell him that I needed his help to find my way. I also didn't fiddle with my purse this time and let the others go ahead before I asked the driver to give me some help.

Therapist: Right, Carol. You did remarkably well that time. If you communicate and handle a problem like this in the future, do you think you'll meet your short- and long-term goals?

Carol: Yeah. I think this way will be better. But I still feel uptight when I'm talking.

Therapist: That's perfectly normal, Carol. When you learn anything new, the first few times feel awkward and stiff. Remember when you first learned how to roller skate, to ride a bike, or drive a car? It takes a lot of practice and success in real-life situations to feel more comfortable and confident. That will come in time, but for the moment, permit yourself to try out these new skills while being somewhat nervous.

Carol: OK, if you say so.

Therapist: Carol, I think you're ready for an assignment to try out what you've learned today with real bus drivers.

Did you notice the therapist's first question after this rerun? It was very carefully phrased to prompt Carol to identify for herself how she improved and to state it publicly. These are directed at generating patients to motivate themselves through "positive self-statement," "positive self-reinforcement," or, less grandly, "blowing your own horn." Getting people to take credit for their accomplishments is often a problem, especially with the chronic and seriously disabled patients we have seen over the years. The tendency to be humble is very strong in most sectors of our society, and patients who have experienced frequent failure are usually very reluctant to give themselves a pat on the back. Learning to describe your accomplishments and then accept the compliments of others, without the "Aw, shucks, tweren't nothin'" response that we have been taught since childhood, takes practice. No one likes a braggart, but no one notices a shrinking violet, either. Taking proper credit is noticed by others—and it often prompts them to give still more compliments.

While getting the patient to speak out and describe his or her progress has an effect on the rest of the group, it will have a profound effect on the patient. The patient will experience what it feels like to say that he or she is successful and that he or she is deserving of praise—and learns the *habit* of thinking of himself or herself that way. The method is very straightforward: Get the person to describe himself or herself as competent and effective and the *feelings* of competence and effectiveness will surely follow. A well-known example of an attempt to do this is the litany led by the Reverend Jesse Jackson when he speaks to young audiences: "I am SOMEBODY!"

You have seen how training steps are intimately interwoven with assessment of the patient's relevant receiving, problem solving, and sending skills. As you gain practice conducting social skills training, the eliciting of assessment information for use in training will become more spontaneous. For neophytes in leading social skills training, however, we recommend a self-conscious and highly structured use of the assessment and training routines. The ways in which training tie in with assessment data are shown in Table 3-10, and we suggest that you frequently refer to it as a means of prompting your own therapeutic skills.

GIVING REAL-LIFE ASSIGNMENTS

The ultimate goal of social skills training is to enable the patient to perform more effectively in the real world. In the mental health arts we frequently find that the patient does well in the hospital, clinic, or office but not so well "outside." This is the problem of generalization—bridging the gap between treatment and the real world. Family, job, school, friendship, and other community-based situations are the crucibles within which the effectiveness of social skills training is tested.

Real-life assignments are the tools we use to overcome this problem of generalization and are intrinsic to social skills training. The assignments allow routine monitoring of progress and, when successfully completed, give the patient a sense of accomplishment that is the best kind of reward. Without an assignment, all the work that went into a training session with the patient is wasted. You'll never know if the skills practiced and apparently learned really have their desired impact in the patient's world. See Table 3-11 for the all-important step of translating

Table 3-10. Intertwining of Assessment With Training in the Teaching of "Receiving," "Processing," and "Sending" Skills

Assessment	Training
"Receiving" Skills	
Who is in scene?	Focus attention and use attentional exercises
Where is situation?	?
What was said?	Prompt correct answers
Who wants what?	Model correct answers
Which emotions were expressed?	Reinforce correct answers
"Processing" Skills	
Define goals, rights, and responsibilities	Adopt a problem-solving set
Generate response alternatives	Prompt, model, and reinforce problem-solving strategies
Anticipate and evaluate consequences	Practice problem-solving through exercises
Choose a response	
"Sending" Skills	
Verbal content	Behavioral rehearsal
Paralinguistic elements	?
Nonverbal components	Modeling
Timing and context	Prompting and cuing
Reciprocity	Positive feedback
	Self-instructions and self-reinforcement
	Practice in vivo

skills learned in the session to a patient's natural environment. Let's see how the therapist gives Carol her homework assignment.

Therapist: Carol, I'd like you to practice getting some information on how to get to destinations from two different bus drivers. I'd like you to stop the number 44 bus and ask how to get to the Sunrise Mall. Because the 44 doesn't go there, you'll have to find out what connections and transfers you'll need to get. Follow the driver's instructions, go to the mall, then stop any bus at the mall, and ask how to get back here. Pay attention to your eye contact and gestures, and remember, you have the right to expect bus drivers to be helpful with travel directions. Take a few deep breaths, and let the air out slowly while you're waiting to get on the bus. That will help you relax. If you want some company while you practice this, ask Karen if she'll go along with you. But Karen would only be there for moral support. Karen, if you go with Carol, pretend you don't know her when the buses stop.

Table 3-11. Step-by-Step Map for Guiding Therapists Through a Typical Session of Social Skills Training Session. The boxed steps represent the application of what has been learned in the session to the patient's real life.

What to Do	How to Do It
1. Give introduction to social skills training.	Welcome patients, introduce yourself, give a brief description of the purpose and methods used in training.
2. Introduce new patients.	Put new patients at ease by asking whether they would prefer being called by their first or last names.
3. Solicit orientation from experienced patients who can explain social skills training to new patients.	Fill in any gaps, if necessary, and select patients to give orientation who are clear, coherent, and upbeat.
4. Reward patients for their contributions to the orientation.	Use praise liberally while looking and smiling at patients.
5. Check homework assignments.	Get details of actual performance, determine obstacles and impediments to generalization, and record results on progress notes.
6. Help each patient pinpoint an interpersonal problem, goal, and scene for this session.	Help patients operationalize their problems by asking what? with whom? where? and when? Watch for problems: face, hands, voice, eyes, loudness, posture.
7. Target scene and interpersonal situation for dry run roleplay.	Help patient select and plan the situation, usually one that recently occurred or that will soon occur; get details for scene from patient.
8. "Set up" the scene.	Enlist others to act as roleplayers with the designated patient, move furniture, get props.
9. Give instructions for the scene.	Collaborate with patient on what should be done, tell roleplaying helpers how to respond, determine the patient's short- and long-term goals from the situation to be rehearsed.
10. Run the scene as a dry run.	Watch patient carefully, looking for deficits and assets in verbal, nonverbal, and paralinguistic elements of the patient's performances; keep the scene brief.
11. Give positive feedback.	Find something to praise, give praise immediately, solicit positive and corrective feedback from other patients, use blackboard or easel to get everyone to participate in giving ratings and feedback.

(continued)

Table 3-11. *Continued*

What to Do	*How to Do It*
12. Assess receiving, processing, sending skills.	Ask the patient these questions: • What did the other person say? • What was the other person feeling? • What were your short-term goals? • What were your long-term goals? • What other alternatives could you use in this situation? • Would one of these alternatives help you reach your goals?
13. Use a model.	Select model for similarity to "real " person in patient's life, be sure patient watches the model performing by annotating the skills being demonstrated.
14. Ensure that patient has assimilated the demonstrated skills.	Ask patient to report on model's performance.
15. Use another model.	Optional, but a good idea if the "real" person in the patient's life might respond unpredictably or with greater resistance than the first model.
16. Give instructions to patient for next rehearsal or rerun.	Concentrate on one or two behaviors that need improvement, ask patient to pinpoint the behaviors that are to be improved.
17. Rerun scene.	Use coaching, including hand signals and whispered prompts and praise as scene unfolds.
18. Give summary positive feedback.	Do it immediately, enlist others to join in praising patient, be specific in praising the improved behavioral elements in the patient's roleplayed performance, use blackboard or easel to point out improvement over earlier performance.
19. Give real-life assignment.	**Make out assignment card, give clear instructions, keep it simple, invite patient to anticipate any obstacles in carrying out the assignment.**
20. Choose another patient for the training sequence and return to step 1.	**Ask for a volunteer first, select someone if no one volunteers.**

Carol, where's your assignment card? I've written down the numbers of the buses, and I've checked off the things I want you to practice. If Karen goes with you, she can sign it to show that you've done your homework.

Carol: All right. You want me to ask directions to a place I already know how to get to?

Therapist: Right. You've done very well here, but now you need practice in the real situation. After you've succeeded asking for directions on routes you're familiar with, you'll try the same thing on unfamiliar routes. That stepwise approach will help build your confidence and your skill level.

Remember the "shaping" principle. Like everything else in social skills training, you should start with easier assignments and gradually increase the difficulty and complexity as the patient's skill and confidence increase. Success and progress can be promoted by constantly adjusting the level of difficulty of the assignments to the changing abilities and level of readiness of the patient. The assignments should follow from the training that has just taken place, and they should be attainable, but just difficult enough to present a challenge. The responsibility for a failed assignment is just as much the therapist's as the patient's.

The importance of setting the level of difficulty to maximize the probability of success can't be overemphasized. The encouragement and applause of the training session will be absent when the patient tries the new skill in the community, and success is a powerful reward that will boost the patient's confidence and willingness to continue to accept more difficult and complex assignments. Setting short-term goals that can be reached in a reasonable time helps the patient to focus on the next little step and the therapist to focus on assignments that will demonstrate that the patient has reached each goal in its turn.

How can you determine the appropriate level of difficulty for an assignment? Your own clinical observations of the patient as he or she interacts during the training session and at other times in natural situations will be an excellent guide. Also, the information you obtain about the patient's capabilities in a wide range of interpersonal situations—from the patient's history and from other informants—can be helpful. But the best clues will come from the patient's cumulative successes and failures in completing assignments given in successive social skills training sessions. One reason for a failed assignment is that it may have been beyond the patient's abilities. More skills training or an easier assignment could solve that problem. In our two decades of experience doing social skills training, we have found that about 60–90 percent of assignments should be completed. If a patient is succeeding more than 90 percent of the time, you can be sure that the assignments are too easy. If the success rate falls below 60 percent, the assignments may be too hard or the training may be focusing on an inappropriate domain that the patient is not ready to tackle.

The therapist should encourage patients to help formulate assignments and should always check out with the patient whether or not he or she feels that the assignment is personally relevant and realistically feasible. Give the patient the option to decline to do an assignment, opting either for a different assignment or for more practice in the training sessions before doing it in real life.

Ask the patient to reflect for a moment on the assignment you describe before you make it final and to tell you and the group if there are any realistic problems that may arise. For example, assigning a patient to ask his social worker to find him a better placement may not be possible if the patient knows that the social worker will be gone on vacation for two weeks. There may be simple, logistical reasons why a patient can't complete an assignment—and you can't always depend on the patient to remember or to volunteer that information.

This process of checking to see if there might be some real obstacles to an assignment can also be used as a time for problem solving. If the need is urgent, waiting for two weeks for the regular social worker may not be wise. Checking with the patient to see if he or she will find out who is filling in for the social worker and opening the subject with that person may be appropriate. If not, then helping him or her explore some ways to make the present living situation more tolerable for the next two weeks would make sense. If you use this approach, you will be a good model of a person who anticipates problems and tries to think out good solutions. Helping the patients see the vagaries of real life in terms of problems that will yield to some planning and analysis is a worthy strategy!

Always prepare patients in advance for the real possibility of failure; in fact, patients should expect to succeed only some of the time with their assignments and not take failure personally. The function of social skills training is to increase the probability that social successes will occur, not to guarantee them. When conducting social skills training in hospitals or other residential care settings, it is advisable to involve the nursing staff or residential managers in the selection and monitoring of assignments. This "programming for generalization" can increase the success rate since the patient's real environment outside the training session will be cued to give reinforcement for even fledgling efforts at using new skills. This also holds true when doing social skills training with children or adolescents. Their parents can fruitfully be involved to promote success experiences with homework.

As the therapist, you may choose to "shape" patients' social effectiveness gradually by repeating assignments several times to consolidate progress and then increase the degree of difficulty in small increments. A good rule of thumb is to "start where the patient is" and then "let the patient's progress be your guide."

The learning principle of "shaping" can be grasped by following the successive assignments set for patients participating in social skills training groups at a community mental health center and VA psychiatric hospital.

Patient: A young man with social and public speaking phobias

Assignment:

1. Introduce himself to three other patients.
2. Give a five-minute "speech" about his weekend activities to a patient group.
3. Go to a city council meeting and ask a question during the discussion period.
4. After the city council meeting, give a three-minute testimonial about the good things that the city offers during the discussion period.

Patient: A 44-year-old man with chronic and disabling obsessive-compulsive disorder

Assignment:

1. Ask a social worker to assist him in finding a nicer boarding home.
2. Describe his positive qualities to a manager of new board-and-care home while applying for entrance.
3. Introduce himself to two other residents at board-and-care home, and give three bits of information about himself; ask for three facts from them at same level of self-disclosure.
4. Call for an appointment with vocational counselor.
5. Request career counseling and job finding help with the counselor.

Patient: A 32-year-old woman with chronic schizophrenia and negative symptoms

Assignment:

1. Have a conversation with a staff member.
2. Talk with the pastor at church.
3. Meet company who visits the family at home.
4. Buy a cake pan in a store.
5. Get a library card.
6. Return a book to the library, pay a fine, and get a new book.
7. Introduce herself to a new neighbor.
8. Introduce herself to one new person, and get personal information from him or her.

9. Go to the library and ask for a particular book.
10. Go to a community center and get a schedule of activities.
11. Talk to the landlord about having some work done.

The assignment should be spelled out in detail and written on a homework card or notebook that the patient carries around. The card itself is a prompt—a reminder to do the homework. A sample assignment card was shown in Figure 3-6. On the reverse side of the card is a handy set of cues reminding the bearer what to do. Finally, the assignment card can serve as a receipt or proof of completion. When signed, it is the patient's badge of courage for having fought the good fight in the cold, cruel world.

PRACTICE EXERCISE

Hewing to a shaping attitude—training skills in small steps that approximate a patient's longer-term goals—is important in the training session as well as in selecting homework assignments. In the following lists, successive, weekly interpersonal goals are given for patients participating in a social skills training group. In each list, one step or subgoal is purposely left vacant. To exercise your own skills in shaping behavior, select an appropriate goal that could lead to successful performance in the patient's real-life situations. There is no single correct answer in this exercise—the point is to select functional, positive, and attainable goals. What would you do if your patient failed to complete the particular goal you selected?

Case 1. A 24-year-old woman with avoidant personality disorder who wanted to make friends and social contacts.

1. Establish eye contact with other group members.
2. Maintain eye contact for 30 seconds with three other group members while they are speaking.
3. Acknowledge job difficulties with boss and request his assistance in learning new tasks.
4. Use conversational "openers" (brief pleasantness) on the beach with strangers.
5. (Fill in this subgoal).
6. Present her positive attributes to prospective employer at job interview.

(continued)

7. Invite two other group members to join her for coffee before group sessions.

Case 2. A 32-year-old single man with schizophrenia who is trying to complete college and attain greater independence from his parents.

1. Discuss vocational aptitude test results and career goals with college counselor.
2. Request tutoring in English composition course from teaching assistant.
3. Initiate study group with two classmates.
4. Request individual therapist to develop a self-control program for him to motivate increased study time.
5. Positively request constructive criticism from his teaching assistant for improving his work in poetry appreciation class.
6. (Fill in a subgoal).
7. Express empathy to his mother who was having conflicts with his older sister.
8. Ask his work supervisor at college library for a promotion.
9. Thank his supervisor for granting him a promotion.
10. Discuss with father his ambivalence about continuing in college versus quitting and getting a full-time job, asking for his father's point of view.
11. Apply to be a volunteer at hospital to work with geriatric patients to test out his interests in a human service occupation.

Case 3. A 58-year-old divorced male who was recently discharged from hospital after recent major depression and who has been abstinent from alcohol abuse for two years. He also is disabled from multiple sclerosis and wants to improve his social life.

1. Ask secretary of Alcoholics Anonymous group to announce his needs for a driver and transportation.
2. Phone at least three agencies and volunteer organizations to advertise his need for a driver.
3. Invite neighbor woman to join him for Thanksgiving dinner.
4. Invite neighbor woman to join him for a coffee date.
5. Phone churches in his locale to acquire information on social and recreational groups and activities.
6. (Fill in a subgoal).
7. Attend senior citizen's program and introduce himself to three strangers.
8. At senior citizen's outing, use open-ended questions to initiate and maintain conversation with two people.

PLOYS FOR GENERALIZATION

While homework assignments are the most widely used method to promote generalization, a few other techniques listed in Table 3-12 should be mentioned. Employing multiple trainers, and training patients to cope with a wide variety of situations, will better simulate the real world and prepare patients for the randomness and uncertainty that exists in their natural environments. If patients have a variety of models to learn from and roleplayers to serve as "targets" for their skills training, they will be better prepared for novelty in their lives. The problem-solving strategy described in this chapter—where patients are coached to generate different alternatives for dealing with interpersonal challenges—provides another technique that can spur generalization. Of course, there's no way that all permutations of situations can be anticipated in the actual training, so giving patients a problem-solving attitude aids readiness for the unexpected.

Bringing the real world into the training session can be a useful ploy. For example, when teaching patients to improve their communication with their relatives, it is always preferable to have their relatives in the session and participating in the roleplays. This not only makes the training more realistic, but it also acquaints the relatives with the goals and purposes of social skills training, thereby enhancing their cooperation with the patient's fledgling efforts. Related to bringing significant others into the training is conducting the training in or near the real-life settings where the patient's social skills must be used. This often requires improvisation and a therapist who is mobile enough to accompany the patient into his social field. Stores, coffee shops, agency offices, parks, recreation centers, and clubs are frequently used sites for in vivo training. Another way to bridge the gap between training sessions and the real world is to "program" the patient's natural environments with supports by others for the patient's initial efforts at using the skills.

Table 3-12. Techniques That Can Be Applied to Promote Generalization of Skills Taught in Social Skills Training to Real-Life Settings

- Homework assignments
- Multiple exemplars and trainers
- Problem-solving strategy
- In vivo practice
- Fading of training structure, frequency, and supervision and reinforcement
- Treatment setting approximates or simulates the "real world"
- Natural reinforcers to support acquired skills
- Skills that are "marketable" and self-sustaining in the community
- Patients to use self-reinforcement
- Repeated practice and overlearning
- Functional and attainable goals in training skills

Mike is a 27-year-old man who had been continuously hospitalized for a year with schizophrenic symptoms that had proven refractory to antipsychotic drugs. He was referred for skills training because of poverty of speech, abject apathy, and social isolation. We introduced Mike to a social skills training program twice weekly for an hour each time. Training goals were to learn how to ask open-ended questions, to give compliments to others, and to use appropriate forms and levels of self-disclosure in conversations. From near-zero levels, Mike increased these conversational skills markedly during "tests" of conversations with the trainer in the training room. However, his level of responding to strangers and others not involved in the training remained nil in the hospital courtyard and dayroom. Only when nursing staff on his unit were instructed to give him occasional prompts and praise for conversing did he show a dramatic increase in generalization. Maintenance of this generalization of conversation was seen at three months after the skills training sessions had ended.

One final technique for helping skills transfer from the training setting into real life should be mentioned, that is, gradually fading the degree of structure in both the training steps and the frequency of the sessions. If the patient is closely coached and abundantly reinforced with continuous praise until the cessation of training, he or she will be ill-prepared to use the skills in natural environments where there is no coaching and where people tend to be stingy about giving praise. Similarly, if training sessions are suddenly terminated after occurring weekly or twice-weekly for months, the patient will suffer "withdrawal" effects from the loss of training. However, if the frequency of the sessions is gradually reduced with increasing intervals for real-life practice, patients will be more likely to keep the skills they have learned. Booster training sessions are always a good idea, especially for seriously mentally disabled patients who may not have a lot of opportunity to practice their newly learned skills. After all, don't we also need booster sessions to keep current and fresh in our professional work?

EVALUATING PROGRESS

You can see how this approach to training social skills relies on checking on performance and progress at every step of the way. The reason should be clear; we want to be sure that what we are doing is working— having some good effect on the patient. But there are some other reasons that may not be so obvious. One has to do with accountability. The time that staff spends with patients is precious. Staff costs make up at least 80 percent of the budgets of most mental health centers, and they seldom spend more than 50 percent of their time on duty in direct contact with patients. Much of what they do is the necessary, often legally required, busy work of running the service. But what the staff *does* with a patient is supposed to be what *changes* or *helps* the patient and prepares the patient to face the world again. So the time is precious, often expressed in the number of staff you are allowed to have working, and many times in terms of taxpayers' money.

Getting the most out of every hour spent with patients makes good sense. And one way of ensuring the survival of your mental health service is being able to show that you and your staff are effective and efficient at what you do.

Finally, no method can remain static for long and survive. As we learn more about the effects of our methods on patients, we can change them, paring away what is not effective, strengthening what is, and adding new and better components. If we are serious about this, then we must become rather compulsive collectors of evidence all along the way. Viewed differently, evaluation needs to be focused on the process, or how well the patient learns the skills during treatment as well as on the outcome, or how well the skills are used outside the clinic. In this case, process evaluation will tell us whether or not social skills were learned in treatment; outcome evaluation will tell us whether the skills generalized to the real world and whether the patient has gained greater social competence.

> Carol's improved *social skills* are reflected by her active participation in the training, in the improved eye contact, and in the positive requests she makes of others. Her increasing *social competence* is shown by her use of public transportation and by the fact that she now holds a volunteer job.

Monitoring Patients' Performances

The best way to determine whether the training is moving along at the best pace is to do frequent progress checks during the behavioral rehearsals. Recording the progress weekly is practical in most settings, especially if the training sessions are held twice a week or more. Otherwise, a note at the end of each session is appropriate. Use a Progress Note or Record Form (see examples in the Appendix), and record both positive and negative aspects of the performance, emphasizing those skills that need further improvement or consolidation. Reviewing these notes will also tell you about which techniques need to be changed or improved. You and your co-therapist can ask yourselves the following questions:

- Are the patient's verbal and nonverbal skills improving at a sufficient rate?
- Does the patient show signs of improved participation in the different parts of the training session?
- Are the patient's goals appropriate? Are they too easy or too difficult?
- Are the methods being used in the training effective with this particular patient?
- Does the patient identify social situations and volunteer to take part in scenes? Or must he or she be prodded and prompted?

This issue of volunteering is particularly important. We have found that the level of spontaneity a patient shows is an excellent indicator of the benefit that patient is receiving. This shouldn't be a surprise to any therapist or educator, since a higher level of involvement is usually a sign that the patient has "bought into" the model and is likely to have learned some of the values and ideas behind it.

On the other hand, continued reluctance to participate, either when called on or spontaneously, points to a number of factors that can be changed. The patient may be extremely anxious or socially inhibited and need special help to feel at ease. The goals may not interest or seem relevant to the patient, which can be remedied by reassessing or renegotiating the goals with the patient. In any case, persistent nonparticipation should be a warning that requires action by the therapist.

Other problems may produce overt signs of discontent with the treatment. Intentional negativism may occur if the patient is moved forward too quickly without being allowed to consolidate the gains that have been made. Additional practice scenes may be necessary to help here.

We have stressed the importance of adopting a philosophy of "shaping" throughout this manual. It may often be necessary to fall back to easier scenes and less demanding situations before moving forward. It is easy to become impatient and want to grasp the gold ring that seems just beyond the patient's reach. As in other therapies, that is a mistake, satisfying the therapist's desires rather than demonstrating the patient's capabilities.

For the persistently negative and noncooperative person, the techniques described in Chapter 5 on Overcoming Resistance to Training may help to break the logjam. Exploring reasons for noncompliance, encouraging ventilation of feelings related to the training, or using paradoxical or "strategic" interventions are often helpful in these difficult cases. Sometimes, the solution is very simple; negative patients may

respond simply by reducing the level of performance expectation temporarily, allowing them to observe other more involved patients practice.
Then, focusing on less personally threatening goals and skills, the therapist may begin to advance the level of difficulty and complexity.

In all cases where progress seems minimal, the patient's goals need to
be reevaluated. Bringing the patient as well as relatives and other caregivers into another planning session will often show that the goals have
to be redefined or that the sequence in which they are addressed needs
to be changed.

Ted was showing difficulty learning how to reestablish friendly relations with his family. He repeatedly practiced roleplay conversations
with his mother and father on the phone without acquiring the desired
positive verbal and nonverbal behaviors. A counseling session revealed
that he really felt a need to establish peer relationships before trying to
repair his relationship with his family, partially because he was afraid of
becoming too dependent on his parents for emotional support.

Monitoring Generalization

The bottom line for effectiveness of social skills training is whether
or not your patient actually uses the skills in real-life situations. The
optimum goal is for the skills to generalize out of the training and into
the patient's daily routine. The skills should be learned so well that they
become a natural part of the patient's behavioral repertoire or, if you
wish, the patient's personality. There are some conditions that have to be
met before this goal can be reached. One we have just covered; the skills
must be learned successfully. Now, when the skill is used by the patient,
it has to meet with a high degree of success, or it will disappear from the
person's repertoire, or personality. It is a well-established finding that
behaviors that are punished or ignored simply disappear. If the skills are
used and are rewarded, it is more likely that they will be used again and
again, until the newly learned social skills become indistinguishable
from those that were learned "naturally." So, keeping track of the success or failure of the patients' real-life assignments will provide you with
the best evidence of the effectiveness of social skills training as therapy.

If you find that the patients' achievements in the training sessions are
not matched by success in real-life assignments, it's time to do some
more troubleshooting. Are the scenes being used in the training good
simulations of the real life? Art must imitate life in social skills training,
not the other way around! The patient may also need more practice in

training or he or she may need to work up to more difficult assignments gradually—the shaping attitude, again. Ask yourself these questions, ask your co-therapists, and above all ask the patients.

Here is an example of a therapist who leads a social skills group discussing a patient with that patient's psychiatrist. Karen, the patient with whom we met earlier, is progressing in the training sessions, but is not reporting enough real-life transfer of her skills.

Therapist: I don't know what Karen's problem is. She's doing fine in the training sessions, but she seems to be having trouble with the assignments.

Psychiatrist: Do you think she's absorbing and internalizing what you've been teaching?

Therapist: Well, she is attentive and conscientious in group, and she does very well using the verbal and nonverbal skills we have been teaching.

Psychiatrist: She may be experiencing more anxiety than she is showing. I know that she has a lot of apprehension about expanding her activities in the real world. Self-assertion and expressing emotions are big issues with Karen. I would recommend taking easy steps, especially for this goal of making friends. Since the assignments represent risks of rejection and fear of failure, easier assignments might produce less anxiety.

Therapist: I agree. We want to give her as many chances as possible to experience success and to reduce her social anxiety. We could try more challenging assignments later on.

For patients who have completed assignments regularly, new goals should be discussed and pinpointed. As a skillful trainer, you will adopt a shaping attitude as you consider the long-term, ultimate goals for your patients. Session by session, you should set smaller goals that lead toward achieving the longer-term goals. Ask yourself,

- For better social adjustment and quality of life (i.e., long-term goals), where should my patient be headed?
- What intermediate steps need to be taken to achieve success in the ultimate (yet feasible) goals? These steps will give you a set of short-term goals.
- How fast should the patient be progressing?

Methods of Monitoring Generalization

Three sources of evaluation are conveniently available for monitoring the progress of patients as they transfer their newly learned (or relearned!) skills to the real world outside the clinic: (1) self-report by the patients, (2) observations of the patients' behavior by others, and (3) the permanent products that are the end results of using social skills. You will recall that we discussed "permanent products" in Chapter 2, and we will briefly summarize their use as it applies to monitoring generalization.

The easiest and least expensive way to evaluate outcome is simply to ask the patient about his or her progress. Patients can give verbal or written descriptions of their experiences in carrying out real-life assignments. Further, they can report on their attempts to use their skills in "new" situations that weren't practiced in the training sessions or used in assignments. A key measure of the reliability of the patient's self-report is the degree and quality of the detailed description of what transpired. You can be more confident that the incident actually occurred if the patient is able to provide a graphic and detailed, blow-by-blow account of "who did what to whom." We have found that patients tell the truth about their assignments more frequently than we had expected. Serious embellishments or distortions are easily spotted by therapists, since it is difficult to maintain them when pressed for supporting details.

If a patient is caught in such a distortion or exaggeration, the therapist should take care to react in a manner that essentially ignores the "lying" issue but emphasizes the possible remedies: reassigning the homework, reassessing the difficulty of the goal, redesigning the homework, or redefining goals. For most patients a moralistic confrontation before an audience could be damaging and might result in the patient dropping out of treatment altogether.

If patients keep a log or diary of real-life experiences that relate to their goals, they are doubly served; recording their successes provides self-reinforcement as well as a means for providing you with a means for monitoring their progress—and adding to the social approval they have already gained. Furthermore, self-monitoring progress helps to heighten the awareness of patients of appropriate situations where they can use their newly acquired skills. Keeping such diaries is common practice in many forms of therapy.

There are different styles and levels of complexity of logs and diaries; thus, if you choose to use this method, your own creativity should be used to tailor the diary to suit the level of sophistication of the patients. Patients can record their progress in terms of the reduction in discomfort they feel as they complete more and more assignments. This can be done by having them estimate their degree of discomfort, tension, or anxiety on a scale of "subjective units of discomfort" that might range from 0 to 100 or 0 to 10. A device to help you and the patient with doing this is the Social Skills Distress Scale, included in the Appendix to this guidebook. Alternatively, scales can be devised that evoke positive ratings of "social confidence."

The diary or logbook method takes more time for everyone than does the self-report approach. It has many advantages, however. It is probably less prone to distortion, but more important, it is tangible evidence of the patient's commitment to the treatment. The diary provides a focus for part of a treatment session. The attention paid to the diary itself by the therapist is attention paid to the patient's increasing efforts toward overcoming the debilitating effects of serious mental disorder.

The behavior of the patient can also be rated directly by an observer and reported back to the therapist. Observers can be family members, friends, or other staff members. The use of other staff as observers is particularly convenient and helpful when the patient is participating in an inpatient, day treatment, or residential care facility, where the behavioral assignments are to be completed in the facility itself. Observers can report on whether or not a patient has actually carried out the assignment as well as rate the outcome, quality, form, and comfort displayed in the interaction.

Finally, the successful completion of homework assignments often produces some type of tangible, permanent product. For example, a depressed housewife, given an assignment to ask her husband to take her out for a social evening, can bring the ticket stubs from the theater or a menu or receipt or business card from the restaurant. A young man with schizophrenia who has been practicing appropriate responses to a job interview can bring to the next session completed job applications and, if eventually successful, a stub from a salary check. Having the "targets" of interpersonal assignments initial or sign the patient's homework cards has already been discussed; it is an excellent way of generating permanent products where none might have existed in the normal course of events. Permanent products are both evidence of progress for the therapist/scientist and symbols of success for a patient.

On a more basic level, they are similar to ages-old methods used to signify prowess. Sending the young adult or initiate on a great quest with a requirement to bring back the feathers of the sacred eagle or the skin of a dangerous animal is well documented in story and song. Gathering trophies and displaying proof of accomplishment have never gone out of style, except with those of us who have been taught that manipulating symbols and concepts is more important than is working with the objects of nature. Returning with the permanent products of success can be a joyful "counting coup" on a frightening and hostile world.

Evaluating Therapists' Skills

At last we come to the "sauce for the goose" part of the evaluation process. Especially during your initial efforts in applying social skills training, you will benefit from self-evaluation and giving yourself positive and corrective feedback to sharpen your competence and the results you are obtaining with the technique. You may wish to consult with a colleague who is already experienced in social skills training, or better still, invite an experienced trainer or behavior therapist to co-lead your individual, family, or group training sessions: Watch their leadership skills and listen to their feedback on your performance. You can use the checklist of therapist competencies in the Practice Exercise at the end of this chapter to guide your self-evaluation.

The questions should be familiar: Are the goals you are setting for your patients realistic, desirable, and functional? Do they serve as small steps leading toward longer-term goals that can yield greater social competence? Are you encouraging inhibited patients to become involved? Did you remember to elicit positive feedback from group members for everyone's rehearsals? How about some of the basic mechanics of the session? Are the practice scenes too long? Do they move along briskly and keep everyone attentive? How are disruptive or evasive behaviors handled? What suggestions can be made for improving future efforts, particularly with challenging patients? In Figure 3-8 you will find a chart outlining the phases that need to be followed and the clinical questions that should be addressed in evaluating the progress of your patients—and your own developing skills as a trainer!

In conclusion, monitoring progress in a systematic way not only benefits your patients, but it will also enable you to accumulate clinical wisdom on the relative effectiveness of different types of training methods with a variety of problems and populations. By multiplying the practice of monitoring and evaluating the efficacy of our methods across all professionals, our field can move ahead, past partisan concerns and artificial boundaries, to evolve even more effective therapy and training techniques. An empirical attitude with a commitment to measuring the results of what we are doing will minimize our attachments to fads and fashions and improve our clinical efforts. And an accumulation of down-to-earth, understandable evidence never hurts when it comes time to stand for your operating budget!

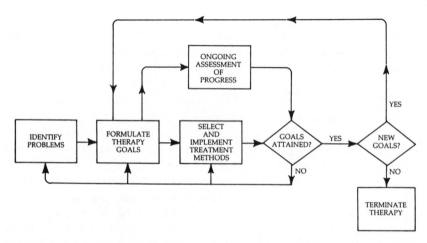

FIGURE 3-8. The process used in behavior therapy, of which social skills training is one example, to monitor therapeutic progress and change and to formulate new goals.

PRACTICE EXERCISES

1. *Planning Guide for Implementing Social Skills Training*   Use the following listing to help you plan your use of social skills training with patients and clients. The value of this guidebook will be multiplied many times if you are successful in applying the methods described to your own clinical work and cases.

a. List four individuals for whom social skills training would be appropriate. These can either be patients that you have primary clinical responsibility for and/or patients with whom you have clinical contact during the week.

b. Of these patients, which one do you think you would most likely be successful with in using the social skills methods? Please write his or her name.

c. What general problem area (e.g., obtaining employment, meeting new friends, talking with a family member) would you choose to work on with this patient?

d. Describe the specific scene and goal that would give this patient a chance to practice this new behavior.

e. At what specific place and at what specific time would you be doing this training?

f. Write out the brief orientation (introduction and purpose) of the session that you would give the patient.

(continued)

g. In what receiving skills is this patient most deficient?

h. In what processing skills is this patient most deficient?

i. What sending behavior(s), verbal or nonverbal, could you most likely be able to reinforce positively after the first dry run of the scene?

j. In what ineffective, extraneous, or distracting behavior(s) would this patient be likely to engage that you could ignore?

k. What behavior(s) could you or someone else model for the patient that he or she could imitate during the second rehearsal of the scene?

l. What realistic "outside the therapy session" assignment could you give the patient, based on his or her performance?

m. Remember to ask for assignment completion information at the next session and to reinforce lavishly assignments that are completed.

2. *Checklist of Competencies for Therapists Conducting Social Skills Training* After you have tried to use social skills training methods with a patient, review the criteria for competence in trainers listed here. Note the clinical skills that you have utilized and those that will need more practice. Return to this checklist frequently as you gain more practice and experience doing social skills training. Reward yourself with praise and other "goodies" for gradually increasing your skill level as a social skills trainer.

_____ Actively helps the patient in setting and eliciting specific interpersonal goals.

_____ Promotes favorable expectations, a therapeutic orientation, and motivation before roleplaying begins.

_____ Assists the patient in building possible scenes by asking "What emotion or communication needs to be expressed?" "Who is the interpersonal target?" and "Where and when will the interaction take place?"

_____ Structures the roleplaying by setting the scene and assigning roles to patient and surrogates.

_____ Engages the patient in behavioral rehearsal—getting the patient to roleplay with others.

_____ Uses self or other group members in modeling more appropriate alternatives for the patient.

(continued)

———— Solicits from the patient, or suggests an alternative behavior for, a problem situation that can be used and practiced during the behavioral rehearsal or roleplaying.

———— Prompts and cues the patient during the roleplaying.

———— Uses an active style of training through coaching, ("shadowing"), being physically out of his or her seat, and closely monitoring and supporting the patient.

———— Gives the patient positive feedback for specific verbal and nonverbal behavioral skills.

———— Identifies the patient's specific verbal and nonverbal behavioral deficits or excesses and suggests constructive alternatives.

———— Ignores or suppresses inappropriate and interfering behavior.

———— Shapes behavioral improvements in small, attainable increments.

———— Evaluates deficits in social perception and problem solving and remediates them.

———— Gives specific, attainable, and functional homework assignments.

SUMMARY

Social skills training works best with groups, but it can be used effectively with individuals or with couples or families. Four to twelve patients in a group is an ideal, but larger groups have been run. A cotherapist is desirable for all groups, but essential for the larger ones. The group setting increases positive expectations, helps with generalization, allows for closer approximation of practice rehearsals to real life, and provides many more opportunities for modeling and learning by imitation. Sessions should last between 45 and 90 minutes and be run as frequently as every day or as little as once a week. Overlearning is both an objective and a training method in this approach.

The structure and fast-pacing of the sessions ensures that behavioral rehearsals will be possible for each patient and that everyone will pay attention. More doing and less talking about what is being done results in a lively pace. Since patients with major psychiatric disorders suffer the equivalent of a learning disability, more effort is needed to keep them engaged. Therapists should be energetic, move around, and be good models for patients to imitate. The therapist is most effective as a teacher of social skills by standing up and moving around to observe and direct the action with a patient.

Television equipment can be used to provide accurate feedback on improvement, as long as it doesn't get in the way of the smooth operation of the group. Positive and corrective feedback is given verbally, although rating can be shown on a flip chart or blackboard to focus attention on which skills are improving. Assignment cards are the only other essential props needed.

Introductions of new patients come first, with a review of the methods and goals of the social skills group done by the leader and veteran group members. The introduction should emphasize the reasons for concentrating on nonverbal behaviors, importance of communicating feelings, and the necessity for homework assignments. Checking on assignments comes next for everyone in the group. The situations that will be practiced for each person come out of this homework review. Then comes the dry run or initial behavioral assessment and rehearsal. Group members practice situations that flow from agreed-upon goals and everyone gets a homework assignment at the end of his or her practice sessions. Scenes are brief because this permits the dissection of complex social situations and the piecing together of small increments of coping skills to achieve long-term goals.

Every scene or situation practiced should include the basic principles of learning: positive feedback in the form of specific approval for effort and accomplishment, models to demonstrate different methods to imitate, shaping by progressing gradually, and extinction of inappropriate behavior by selective inattention. Along with the nonverbal elements of communication, social perception and problem-solving skills are targeted in sessions. Receiving, processing, and sending skills can be tested and demonstrated in each practice by using questions designed for this purpose. Coaching by whispering instructions, using a set of standard hand signals and even physically prompting patients during rehearsals all help elicit the best possible performance in repeated practice efforts. Praise by the therapist and the others in the group serves as the method for maintaining motivation and interest. As the training moves along, patients are trained to make positive self-statements so that they can provide their own positive feedback away from the group setting.

Giving real-life assignments is essential for generalizing skills form the rehearsal to the real world. They also help monitor how well the patient has learned social perception and problem-solving skills. Assignments give the opportunity for risk of failure as well as for the best kind of reward: a sense of accomplishment. Generalization can be enhanced by using several different trainers, and a variety of models. Bringing the real world into the training can be done by inviting family members to participate or by taking the patient out into the actual situation. As progress is made, the high degree of structure inherent in this method, as well as the frequency of the sessions, should be "faded" or gradually reduced. *PROGRESS*

Evaluation of how each group is progressing is essential for therapists and administrators alike. Planning for future groups and justifying requests for resources demand an accounting of outcome. Social skills training lends itself to gathering outcome data. Monitoring each patient's progress in learning the skills and achieving goals should be done weekly, and the effectiveness of generalization of training for each patient should be recorded when the assignments are checked. Self-report, observations by others, and collecting permanent products can all be used to document how effective the training has been.

Spending time individually with patients ensures their involvement and participation in setting long- and short-term goals. Concrete, personal goal examples from the therapist help patients to understand how to set their own appropriate goals. Doing a "dry run" or "on-line" assessment by staging a roleplay of a problem situation can also clarify the types of goals to work toward. Getting the patient to describe the real situation in detail requires asking "who?" "what?" "when?" and "how?" It is vital to keep each training sequence brief and well-paced. Keep moving around, don't sit down while the action is going on. Observe the behavior of the patient carefully in the roleplay simulations of real-life situations to check the goals you and the patient have chosen.

Chapter 4
Friendship and Dating Skills

The first three chapters of this guidebook have familiarized you with the fundamentals of social skills training, including assessment and training strategies for teaching a wide range of skills to psychiatric patients. Now we will focus on a social skills group designed to enhance functioning in one specific interpersonal area—*friendship and dating*. The impoverished quality of life of many chronic psychiatric patients is nowhere more evident than when one observes their lack of social support, companionship, and friendly interactions with others in their living environments, whether at home, in the hospital, day treatment center, community rehabilitation program, or social center. Even patients who are comparatively well adjusted, such as those who are able to work or who have adequate independent living skills, often complain of the loneliness and isolation they experience by being alienated from family and not having friends. When they attempt to reach out they encounter difficulties initiating new relationships.

The tendency for persons with a psychiatric illness, such as schizophrenia or depression, to avoid unfamiliar people and situations reduces their opportunities to establish meaningful friendships and hampers them from forming relationships with members of the opposite sex. Nevertheless, making friends and relating to the opposite sex are important goals for most patients who, while lacking know-how and initiative, are highly motivated to acquire the skills crucial to achieving such goals.

In addition to enhancing the quality of life by deepening patients' interpersonal relationships, dating and friendship skills may improve the outcome of long-term mental illnesses by broadening patients' social support networks and providing greater resources for buffering the negative effects of stress. Premorbid social and sexual adjustment have long been known to be potent predictors of the course of psychiatric disorders. For many patients, learning friendship and dating skills will further their social development that was arrested at the onset of their illness.

137

SOCIAL SKILLS MODULES

In this chapter, a method for teaching friendship and dating skills is organized as a module for inserting into existing psychiatric treatment programs. A module consists of a trainer's manual, a patient's workbook, and a demonstration video for modeling the knowledge and skills required for community adaptation. A series of skills modules for training social and independent living has been designed at the UCLA–Brentwood VA Clinical Research Center for Schizophrenia and Psychiatric Rehabilitation. They include training in Medication Self-management, Conversation Skills, Recreation for Leisure, Symptom Self-management, and Grooming and Self-care. The main advantage of the modular format is that patients can be assigned to social skills groups depending on their specific behavioral deficits.

Each module provides training in a few skill areas, which when learned in combination, result in effective social performance. Each skill area is composed of a number of component skills. For example, one skill area taught in the Friendship and Dating module is "Making Friends," which includes three component skills: giving compliments, receiving compliments, and finding activities to do together. Component skills are taught using the procedures described in Chapter 3, but in a systematic sequence of learning activities as shown in Figure 4-1. A heavy emphasis is placed in the instructional methods on interpersonal problem solving, homework assignments, and in vivo exercises. Skill areas build on one another, and hence are taught in a specific sequence. Patients must master all the component skills in a given skill area before they proceed to learn the components of the next skill area. By the end of a module, patients have acquired all the component skills included in each of the skill areas and are ready to use them in their daily routine.

Problem-Solving Training

Patients learning new social skills often encounter unexpected obstacles when attempting to use these skills in novel situations. As a result, patients may not achieve their goals and may become discouraged and give up. To minimize these frustrations, intensive training in solving common problems that prevent patients from attaining their goals is included as a feature of skills-training modules. Specific obstacles are identified and problem-solving training is conducted for each skill area of a module. Training in problem solving is conducted following a five-step model including definition of the problem, generation of possible alternative solutions, evaluation of each alter-

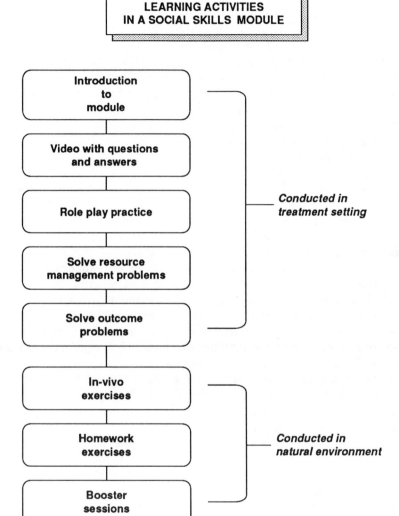

**LEARNING ACTIVITIES
IN A SOCIAL SKILLS MODULE**

Introduction
to
module

Video with questions
and answers

Role play practice

Solve resource
management problems

Solve outcome
problems

*Conducted in
treatment setting*

In-vivo
exercises

Homework
exercises

Booster
sessions

*Conducted in
natural environment*

Figure 4-1. The Sequence of Learning Activities Which Are Used to Teach the Component Skills in Each Module.

native, selection of the best alternative, and planning how to implement the alternative selected.

Interwoven throughout the specific skills included in each module, training is given to patients in overcoming two types of obstacles: "resource management problems" and "outcome problems." Solving resource management problems requires patients to anticipate and gather the resources necessary to implement a particular social skill. For example, if an individual has the verbal skills necessary to ask another person out on a date, he or she may first need to have specific resources such as suitable attire, money, and transportation.

Training in solving outcome problems is designed to help patients identify alternative response options when people in the environment do not respond in accordance with the expected and desired outcome. For example, if an individual suggests to an acquaintance that they do an activity together and the acquaintance rejects the offer, what alternatives does the individual have for achieving the goal of sharing an activity with another person?

Setting the Stage

The Friendship and Dating module can be taught to individual patients or in groups. The training should be conducted at least once a week, and preferably more frequently since massed practice (i.e., frequent sessions over a brief period of time) is a superior means of learning new skills. Three sessions per week is an optimal frequency since it allows one day between sessions for the completion of homework assignments. Session length should be between one and one-and-a-half hours. Depending on the frequency of sessions, group size, and the level of functioning of the participating patients, the module can take between two and four months to complete.

The only equipment required for the group is a blackboard or flipchart for listing reasons for learning a particular skill, displaying the specific skill components, and showing the problem-solving steps. A video-recorder, camera, and monitor can be useful for modeling the targeted skills and providing video feedback to patients after roleplaying, but it is not essential. If video equipment is not utilized, however, two group leaders are recommended to provide "person power" to model the desired skills in well-planned roleplays.

The group can be conducted in a variety of settings, including psychiatric hospitals, outpatient clinics, day treatment centers, community residential programs, community mental health centers, and psychosocial clubs for the chronically mentally ill. With the emphasis on making friends and finding companionship, even patients residing in long-term institutions may benefit from the module.

Patient Selection

Patients participating in this module should have a minimum of psychotic symptoms and be able to maintain their attention for the duration of the 60- to 90-minute session. Entry criteria for patients also include competence in basic conversational skills (e.g., eye contact, voice loudness, fluency, appropriate affect) and adequate self-care skills (e.g., grooming and hygiene). Without these essential social "building blocks," even patients who acquire the behaviors taught in the Friendship and Dating module are doomed to failure when others find them unpleasant to interact with. Thus, social skills training for more basic skills is often necessary to prepare patients to participate in the Friendship and Dating module. The prospect of learning friendship-making skills can serve as an incentive in motivating patients to participate in acquiring the prerequisite basic skills.

Useful assessment information in preparing for a patient's entry into this module can be obtained through a brief interview with the patient, discussions with significant others, and roleplay tests. For example, the following questions can help you determine whether a patient will benefit from this module:

- Is the person able to initiate, maintain, and end conversations with unfamiliar people?
- Can the person accurately recognize emotions in other people?
- Can the person express positive feelings to others?
- Does the patient have any friends?
- Is the person comfortable when interacting with members of the opposite sex?
- Has the person dated other people recently?

These questions provide useful general information about friendship and dating patterns and target areas for modification. More precise behavioral assessment of each patient's assets, deficits, and inappropriate behaviors can be obtained from roleplay tests. By employing a standard set of roleplay scenarios, patients' performances can be compared with each other, and their individual progress can be assessed over time.

The roleplay should be acted out with one patient at a time and a staff member playing the part of the other person in the scene. The interaction should be relatively brief, between 30 seconds and 2 minutes, and ideally should be audio- or videotaped for subsequent rating and replay for feedback. The roleplay scenario is read to the patient, who is instructed to act as though he or she were actually in that situation. Since many psychiatric patients have difficulty in accurately following verbal instructions, ask the following questions before beginning the roleplay to confirm that the patient has understood the situation.

Therapist: What is my role in this scene?
Patient: You're another patient at my day treatment center.
Therapist: What is your task in this roleplay?
Patient: To start a conversation with you.
Therapist: Great! Let's get started.

The patient should be praised for positive aspects of his or her role-play performance and encouraged when rough spots are encountered. Examples of roleplay scenarios that assess skills taught in the Friendship and Dating module are shown in Table 4-1.

SKILL AREAS

The Friendship and Dating module is divided into four skill areas, which are taught in sequence, each skill area building on the ones taught before:

- Initiating conversations with strangers
- Recognizing and expressing emotions
- Making friends
- Going on a date

INITIATING CONVERSATIONS WITH STRANGERS

The first skill area focuses on interacting with relatively unfamiliar people; identifying and following through on conversational topics, attentive listening, and gracefully exiting conversations are important skills mastered in this area.

Psychiatric patients often misjudge others' emotions and have difficulty expressing or modulating their own feelings. The ability to recognize and express emotions accurately is critical to forming and deepening interpersonal relationships. Mastery of this skill area enables patients to assess others' feelings toward their own behavior and evaluate others as prospective friends.

Friendship is the mutual enjoyment of companionship, usually to the point of desiring and arranging repeated get-togethers. Complimenting the other person and expressing affection are skills that make others feel good, and usually make us more pleasant to be around. Additional skills that facilitate the making of friends include gradually becoming more self-disclosing, choosing activities to do together, and compromising and negotiating with the other person.

To be successful in dating, one must be able to plan and follow through a date with a member of the opposite sex. Repeated dating with one other person requires skills in intimacy and good communication.

Table 4-1. Roleplay Assessment Scenarios for Friendship and Dating Module

1. You are waiting to catch a bus you take to your day treatment center every day. You notice a woman (man) sitting on the bench opposite you who you have seen waiting there on several earlier occasions. She (he) is alone, and you would like to start a conversation with her (him). You go up to her (him) and say . . .

2. You have been participating in a recreation group that meets once a week to do leisure activities such as bowling and swimming. Two weeks ago a new patient joined the group, but you have not spoken to her (him) yet. This morning you decide you would like to start a conversation with him (her), so you sit next to her (him) on the van on the way to go bowling. You say . . .

3. Somebody you know from your boarding home has just bought a bucket of Kentucky Fried Chicken and offers to share it with you. He (she) says, "Hey want to dig into some fried chicken?" You respond . . .

4. A friend of yours has just bought a new denim jacket, and you like the way it looks on him (her). You say . . .

5. You would like to go to the movie with a friend of yours tonight. Your friend says he (she) would prefer to go out to dinner. You really want to see the movie, so in response you say . . .

6. A friend of yours just got back from seeing an exhibit at a museum, and you would like to find out more about it and your friend's reaction to it. Your friend says, "I went to an exhibit at the natural history museum today." In response, you say . . .

7. A friend of yours has just confided in you about a family conflict he (she) has been having. Your friend appreciates being able to talk to you about this, and you would like to tell him (her) how you feel about your friendship with him (her). Your friend says, "You know, I'm really glad I could talk this over with you. I really feel comfortable talking with you." You say . . .

8. Over the past several weeks you have talked a number of times with a woman (man) at your day treatment program. You would like to ask this person to join you on a date. You are both sitting in the lounge at the day program before activities have begun, and you notice that she (he) is casually reading the newspaper. You go up to her (him) and say . . .

9. You have been on your first date with a man (woman) you have known for several weeks. You have come back from seeing a movie together, and you have enjoyed spending the time with this person. You are about to go back to your own apartment now and would like to end the date by telling the person what you thought of the evening. You say . . .

The specific component behaviors taught in "Making Friends" and "Going on a Date" skill areas are displayed in outline form in Table 4-2.

To illustrate the process of teaching the Friendship and Dating module, we will follow the progress of the same group of patients introduced in the previous chapters: Ted, Karen, Carol, and Allen. Since friendship and dating skills build on more basic skills, we will assume that these patients, particularly Allen and Karen, have improved upon some of their basic conversational skills by participating in the basic social skills training group described earlier. Allen has continued to be rather quiet and rarely initiates conversations. However, his eye contact has improved, he speaks more clearly and with a firm voice tone, and he is better able to stay on the conversational topic. Karen still occasionally complains of feeling anxious, but this has improved with roleplay prac-

Table 4-2. Component Social Skills for "Making Friends" and "Going on a Date" Skill Areas

"Making Friends"

A. Matching level of self-disclosure with other person (low-medium-high level of self-disclosure)

B. Giving compliments
1. Look at person
2. Tell what you like about them: be specific
3. Use a positive voice tone and facial expression

C. Receiving compliments
1. Look at person
2. Thank him or her
3. Acknowledge the compliment by
   a. Saying how it makes you feel, or
   b. Saying how you feel about the item that was complimented

D. Compromising and negotiation
1. State your viewpoint
2. Listen to the other person's viewpoint
3. Repeat back what you heard
4. Suggest a compromise

E. Finding activities to do together
1. Tell other person your interests
2. Ask about his or her interests
3. Identify similar or common interests you have
4. Suggest an activity to do together

F. Expressing affection
1. Choose a time and place when you can talk with the other person in private
2. Judge if person appears interested
3. Express affection in warm, caring voice tone
4. Tell person why you feel this way

"Going on a Date"

A. Enhancing physical attractiveness
1. Grooming and hygiene
2. Appropriate attire
3. Pleasant facial expression and warm voice tone

B. Asking for a date
1. Choose an appropriate person to ask
   a. Someone you are acquainted with
   b. Someone potentially available (i.e., who does not have a partner)
   c. (Optional) Someone of comparable age and status (e.g., not a staff member)
2. Judge if person is available to discuss the invitation
3. Suggest an activity to do together
   a. Think of an activity, date, time, and meeting place before asking
   b. Be positive, for example, "How would you like to . . . " rather than "You wouldn't like to . . . with me?"
4. Be willing to compromise and negotiate when deciding where to go on a date

C. Handling uncomfortable silences
1. Judge if person appears uncomfortable

(continued)

Table 4-2. *Continued*

   2. Say something
      a. Start a new topic
      b. State a preference
      c. Ask person an open-ended question
      d. Compliment the person
   D. Ending a date
      1. Tell person you enjoyed being with him or her
      2. Tell person you would like to see him or her again (if true)
      3. Kiss person or shake hands if appropriate (optional)
      4. Say good-bye/good night

tice and in vivo exercises. In addition, she does not appear as nervous as before and is motivated to improve her skills when interacting with men.

INTRODUCTORY LEARNING ACTIVITY

The group meets twice a week for an hour-and-a-half at the local community mental health center and is being run by one leader. We join the group at the beginning of the introductory session and initial learning activity, which is aimed at clarifying the goals, purpose, and benefits of participating in the module.

Therapist: I'm glad that we're all here now for the first session. I'd like to begin by discussing the goal of this group, which is to improve your skills in making friends and dating. Before we talk about what some of those skills are, I'd like to hear from each of you about why this is an important goal.

Ted: Isn't that an obvious question?

Therapist: Perhaps, but each person is a little different and has his or her own ideas. Ted, why do *you* think it's important to be able to make friends?

Ted: Maybe I could find someone to hang out with.

Therapist: That's a good reason. It's enjoyable to spend time with another person. (Therapist writes down this reason on blackboard, and subsequent reasons as they are generated.)

   Can anyone think of another benefit of having friends or dating?

Karen: (After a pause) Well, when you have a friend you have someone you can talk to when you feel down or upset—

Ted: —or mad!

Therapist: That's right! It's nice to have someone to confide in, whether we're feeling bad or when we have good feelings too. In fact, we know that having a confidante can reduce your risk of getting depressed. Carol, can you think of another advantage of being able to make friends?

Carol: Uhh, I don't know. (Pause) To do things with?

Therapist: Yes. Would you agree with that, Allen?

Allen: I guess so.

Therapist: Allen, what would be an example of something you could do with a friend?

Allen: Listen to records.

Therapist: Good idea! I think we've come up with some real good reasons to be able to make friends. Making friends is a goal that can be achieved by learning several skill areas, which we will focus on in this group. The most basic of these skill areas is knowing how to start conversations with strangers. Before you can make friends with a person, you need to get to know the person by exchanging information and experiences. That's what we are going to start working on today.

Notice how the therapist elicited the rationale for the module from the patients by asking specific questions and drawing everyone into the discussion. Encouraging patients to verbalize the advantages and values of the module's skills enhances their motivation to attend sessions and learn the component behaviors. The relevance of each component skill to the patients' long-term goal of making friends and dating must also be clearly articulated during the introductory learning activity.

ROLEPLAY LEARNING ACTIVITY

We join our group again the following week, after two sessions devoted to watching demonstrations and practicing how to start conversations. Specific skills that have been shown on video and through "live" demonstrations by the therapist included samples of superficial but affable greetings and conversational openers—while making eye contact and having a pleasant facial expression. Colloquial expressions are highlighted, especially those that can serve as frequent exchanges at times of encountering friends or acquaintances—"What's happening?" "How are you doing?" and "Have a nice day!" The present session has been in progress for about 20 minutes, and the therapist has guided several patients through roleplays of initiating two conversations, one with an unfamiliar person and one with a familiar person. The therapist has introduced "active verbal listening skills" as the focus of today's session.

The dialogue picks up where the therapist begins to describe the distinction between open-ended and closed-ended questions.

Therapist: Another important active listening skill is asking questions. Asking good questions can really keep the conversation flowing and is a way of showing the other person that you're interested in what they have to say. Let's say someone you know just told you that he saw the movie *Gone with the Wind*. What's an example of a question you could ask about the movie?

Carol: Who starred in it?

Therapist: Good! Who can think of another question to ask?

Allen: (Softly) Where was the movie playing?

Therapist: That's another good question, Allen. Ted, can you think of another question you could ask?

Ted: What did you like best in the movie?

Therapist: Yes, you could find out what the person liked in the movie. When asking questions, there are two general types of questions you can ask: "open-ended" questions and "closed-ended" questions. A closed-ended question can be answered with a "Yes" or a "No" or a single word, but an open-ended question is better at producing a longer response from the other person. (Therapist writes definitions on the blackboard.) Carol, is the question "Did you like the movie?" an open-ended or closed-ended question?

Carol: Uh, I don't know.

Therapist: What was the question we are considering?

Carol: "Did you like the movie?"

Therapist: Right! Can that be answered with a yes or a no? (Points to blackboard)

Carol: Yes, it can. That makes it a closed-ended question.

Therapist: Exactly. Let's practice with a couple more questions. How about the question, "What did you like best in the movie?" Is it open- or closed-ended?

Ted: Open-ended.

Therapist: How did you know that?

Ted: Because it can't be answered with a yes or a no.

Therapist: Right!

(The therapist provides several more examples for patients to discriminate between open- and closed-ended questions. Following this, the therapist structures a roleplay for patients to rehearse the conversation skills.)

Therapist: Let's do a roleplay to practice these conversation skills. Karen, I'd like to start with you.

Karen: What do I have to do?

Therapist: You are going to listen actively to someone tell you about something and then ask an open-ended question. The goal is to make the other person understand you are interested in what they are saying. Who has an experience they would like to describe to Karen? For example, tell her something you've done recently that you could talk about for a couple of minutes.

Carol: I could tell her about a trip I took over the weekend.

Therapist: That's a good idea. (Chairs are rearranged so that Carol and Karen face each other.) Carol, I'd like you to describe to Karen some of the interesting things you did or saw on your trip. Karen, your job is to practice your listening skills; that is, saying "uh huh," paraphrasing, and asking questions to find out about Carol's trip. Ask as many open-ended questions as you can, because they help keep the other person talking. Let's review your roles in this scene. Carol, what are you going to do?

Carol: Tell Karen about my trip.

Therapist: And, Karen, what's your role?

Karen: To show Carol that I'm listening to her and to ask open-ended questions.

Therapist: Very good. I'd like the other group members to watch Karen carefully and to count how many open-ended questions she asks. Okay?

Ted & Allen: Okay.

(Carol and Karen settle into their chairs to begin.)

Carol: I went on a little shopping trip last Saturday with my parents. (Pause)

Karen: Uh huh.

Carol: We went down to the Italian market.

Karen: Uh huh. (Pause)

Therapist: (Whispering to Karen) Ask what she bought.

Karen: What did you buy?

Carol: All sorts of things. Like pasta and some strawberries.

(Therapist points to "open-ended questions" on the blackboard for Karen.)

Karen: How do you like to fix and eat pasta?

Carol: With vegetables and tomato sauce.

Karen: That sounds really tasty and nutritious, too. It must be fun to go shopping at the Italian market. What kinds of stalls do they have there?

Carol: Mostly food, but they also sell some clothes and crafts and there's even a fortune-teller there.

Therapist: Let's stop here. Karen, you did a nice job finding out about Carol's trip. (Turning to Ted and Allen) What active listening skills did you notice Karen using just then?

At this point, the therapist elicits specific positive feedback about Karen's performance and proceeds to engage the other group members in similar rehearsals. This sample dialogue illustrates the typical flow of skills training in the roleplay learning activity of a module.

Over the following several weeks the group focuses on improving conversational skills, with homework assignments gradually requiring longer conversations, with less familiar persons, and with members of the opposite sex. Karen has reported she experiences less anxiety when conversing, and even Allen, who continues to be quiet, is more fluent and able to identify suitable conversational topics.

"RECOGNIZING AND EXPRESSING EMOTIONS" SKILL AREA

The group has now moved on to the second skill area, "Recognizing and Expressing Emotions." In the introductory learning activity the patients identify the importance of accurately recognizing others' emotions; for example, by gauging the other's reaction to what is being said, a socially perceptive person can elect to either continue, change topics, or end the conversation. Next, in the modeling learning activity, patients observe videotaped actors demonstrating key emotions and become sensitive to vocal tone and facial cues. The therapist engages the patients in an exercise to improve their ability to recognize and express emotions nonverbally (i.e., facial expression) and paralinguistically (i.e., speech tone). To do this exercise, the therapist prepares a set of at least 20 index cards, each containing three elements: (1) a single sentence describing a specific event with emotional overtones, (2) one of five emotions potentially relevant to the event (pleasant, interested, angry, bored, and sad), and (3) a quotation by a speaker describing the situation. Some examples are

- Your dog just died. (sad) "My dog just died."
- You are sitting on the beach listening to the waves. (pleasant) "It's really nice to be relaxing here on the beach."
- Your friend is 45 minutes late. (angry) "What took you so long?"

- A friend just saw a movie you would like to see. (interested) "I've been wanting to see that movie. What's it like?"
- A neighbor is telling you about his car and you're only listening to be polite. (bored) "I'm really not that interested in hearing about the car."

The goal of the exercise is for the participants to practice recognizing the emotions communicated by others and to learn to express their own emotions more clearly. After shuffling the deck of cards, the first group member selects the top card and reads it to himself or herself. The person is instructed to imagine he or she is in the situation and to convey the specific emotion *using facial expressions only*. The other group members try to identify which emotion is being expressed. To be sure that all group members have the opportunity to identify different emotions, the therapist may ask individual members to discriminate the emotion. Inaccurate recognition of emotions may be due to poor sending skills by the person conveying the emotion, poor social perception skills by the viewer, or both. If several group members fail to recognize the emotion, then the sender is given feedback to improve its clarity, and the expression is repeated. For example, smiling enhances pleasantness, raising eyebrows expresses interest, a frown communicates sadness, a scrunched-up nose and glaring signify anger, and lowered averted eyes suggest boredom.

Allen had particular difficulty accurately recognizing and expressing emotions nonverbally in this exercise. He sometimes mistook the interested facial expression for the pleasant one (or vice versa) and had trouble discriminating sad, angry, and bored from each other consistently. Furthermore, others felt he conveyed boredom when he intended to express other emotions instead. You can see here how the therapist shapes Allen's skills at communicating emotions nonverbally. Allen has just tried to portray an angry facial expression for the card describing a friend who is late for an appointment.

Therapist: Okay, Allen, that was a good effort. Carol, can you tell which of the five emotions Allen was expressing?

Carol: I'm not sure.

Therapist: Try and guess.

Carol: Are you feeling bored, Allen?

Allen: Uh, no. I'm supposed to feel mad.

Therapist: Karen and Ted, could you help us out here? Do you agree with Carol that Allen looked bored?

Ted: I thought he looked a little bored, but maybe a little pissed off too. Anyway, he sure didn't look too happy!

Karen: I think so too, but it was hard to tell what he was feeling.

Therapist: That's very helpful. I'd like us to give some even more specific feedback to Allen to help him improve his facial expressiveness. Carol, what made Allen look bored rather than angry?

Carol: Well, he didn't look at me very much, so I thought he wasn't interested.

Therapist: Good. Do you have anything to add, Ted or Karen?

Ted: Wrinkle up your nose and squint if you want to look mad, like this!

Therapist: That's very good feedback, Ted. Allen, try scrunching up your nose like Ted. (Allen imitates Ted.)

Therapist: Good. Now, I'd like you to try another situation, Allen, and this time scrunch up your nose, and look right at Carol. Okay?

Allen: I feel uncomfortable when I look right at someone's eyes.

Therapist: Sometimes it helps to look near, but not right at the person's eyes, like at their nose or forehead. (Therapist selects a different card with an angry scene and gives it to Allen.)

Allen: Okay, I'll try it again . . .

This time Allen's performance is significantly better, and he receives abundant praise from the other group members. In addition, his tendency to avoid eye contact and avert his gaze when interacting with others impaired his ability to recognize others facial expressions accurately. With more practice, and monitoring his gaze when looking at others (such as providing a prearranged signal to Allen when he looked away), Allen's ability to recognize facial expressions steadily improved.

After the group members have practiced recognizing and expressing facial expressions, the exercise is repeated with participants practicing both nonverbal and paralinguistic emotion cues. The goal here is to integrate facial expression and voice tone recognition and to ensure that these two communicative channels are expressed consistently with each other.

The initial component skills trained in this skill area involve nonverbal and paralinguistic features of emotion recognition. When patients have demonstrated competence in these skills, verbal skills relevant to the communication of feelings and preferences are taught. The final educational objective in the skill area of "Recognizing and Expressing Emotions" is shifting topics during a conversation. This ability requires competence in initiating and maintaining a conversation, as well as accurate recognition of subtle changes in the other person's emotions. Changes in a conversational partner's emotions can provide valuable information about whether to continue with a topic (interest), shift topics (boredom), or end the conversation. Shifting topics is taught in roleplays in which the "partner" is privately instructed by the therapist to shift to a designated emotion during the enacted conversation, and the rehearsing patient must determine how to respond.

"MAKING FRIENDS" SKILL AREA

The next skill area is "Making Friends," which includes monitoring levels of self-disclosure, a range of affiliative behaviors (e.g., giving compliments, expressing affection), and identifying and organizing activities to do with someone else. Matching the other person's level of self-disclosure with that of your own, and disclosing personal information gradually are important skills in making friends, since prematurely high self-disclosure can make people feel uncomfortable. Teaching patients to match the self-disclosure level of another person requires, first, that they be able to recognize different levels of self-disclosure from the other person and, second, that they be able to offer similar levels themselves.

Patients are taught to recognize three different levels of self-disclosure: low, medium, high. After clarifying and discussing the importance of self-disclosure from the group members, the therapist provides examples of self-disclosure for patients to discriminate among. For example, the following statements are demonstrated by the therapist who, through questions and answers, teaches patients to discriminate among the three levels of self-disclosure.

Low
- "I live in an apartment around the corner."
- "I like to eat breakfast at McDonald's."

Medium
- "I go to church regularly."
- "I like horror films."

High
- "I got into an argument yesterday with my mother and feel upset about it."
- "I believe in reincarnation."

Following practice at identifying levels of self-disclosure, roleplays are structured for patients to rehearse matching their levels of self-disclosure. For example, Ted began a conversation with Carol at a low level of self-disclosure, telling her about a movie he saw and liked. After she acknowledged her own interests in movies, Ted moved to a medium level of self-disclosure by telling Carol that he wished he had more money to visit the Universal Studios tour. Carol responded that she enjoyed that tour several years ago, but would like to go again. Then, moving to a high level of self-disclosure, Ted expressed a desire to take Carol on a date there.

As we join our group again in the module, the members have become more competent at identifying and conveying emotions and are able to discriminate different levels of self-disclosure. Earlier in today's session, Carol shared with the group that she sometimes reveals too much about herself early in conversations with people, who then tend to avoid or reject her. She is eager to practice matching her level of self-disclosure with the other person in a roleplay, and Ted has agreed to play her acquaintance.

Therapist: Carol, what's your goal in this roleplay?

Carol: To have a nice, little conversation and not reveal too much about myself.

Therapist: Right. Ted, let's pretend that you've met Carol a few times before, but you don't know each other very well. It's lunch-time right now, and you choose a seat next to Carol. I'd like you to start the conversation at a low level of self-disclosure, and then work up to a medium level. Okay?

Ted: All right.

(Chairs are rearranged so that Ted and Carol face each other, with a table placed between them.)

Ted: I think the food here stinks. What do you think?

Carol: Oh, it's not so bad, and you can't beat the price.

Ted: That's true, it's cheap. Actually, I kind of like it when they make those special pasta dishes, like fettucini Alfredo.

Carol: I go for the roasted chicken.

Ted: It's so crowded, though. Crowds make me feel uncomfortable.

Carol: I know what you mean. I don't mind crowds, but I'm afraid of high places, so it's kind of the same thing.

Therapist: Let's stop here. You did a nice job in that roleplay, Carol. And, Ted, you helped keep the ball rolling. Karen, at the beginning of the conversation, what was Ted talking about and what level of self-disclosure was he at?

Karen: He talked about the food. I guess that's pretty low in self-disclosure.

Therapist: I agree. Allen, did Carol match Ted's low level of self-disclosure at the beginning?

Allen: I think so. She talked about food too.

Therapist: Right. How about later in the conversation? Did Ted reveal more about himself?

Karen: Yes, he talked about not liking crowds.
Therapist: Yes he did. Ted, did Carol match your medium level of self-disclosure?
Ted: She told me about being afraid of heights. We were pretty closely matched, I'd say . . .

Notice that the therapist provided fairly detailed instructions to Ted about what level of self-disclosure to portray. With another less verbal patient, the therapist might also have suggested some possible topics for self-disclosure. Carol performed very well in the roleplay, not only matching her level of self-disclosure to Ted's, but also converging on the same topics (i.e., food preferences and fears). Teaching patients to monitor their own levels of self-disclosure can be facilitated by having them construct a list of self-disclosures that they rate along the low-medium-high dimension.

"GOING ON A DATE" SKILL AREA

The group has been meeting for another five weeks, during which time they have covered the rest of the "Making Friends" skill area and have started on the "Going on a Date" skill area. The first educational objective in this skill area is to learn methods for enhancing physical attractiveness. Patients are informed that physical attractiveness has consistently been found to be an important factor in determining how desirable a person is for dating. However, contrary to popular belief, there are steps people can take to make themselves more attractive to others. Not only are grooming and personal hygiene important to creating an attractive appearance, but so are the verbal and nonverbal skills people use when interacting with others. A pleasant facial expression, voice tone, and inflection also can contribute to attractiveness.

LEARNING ACTIVITIES FOR SOLVING PROBLEMS

When we join the Friendship and Dating module again, one session has been spent working on strategies for enhancing physical attractiveness and two sessions on asking a person out on a date. Patients are now ready to be taught to solve resource problems and outcome problems related to dating. Anticipating the resources necessary to use their social skills and identifying alternative behaviors if goals are not achieved maximizes the chances that patients' best efforts will meet with successful outcomes. The problem-solving approach to evaluating resource needs when asking a person out on a date is illustrated with Ted, who has learned dating skills rapidly, but tends to become easily frustrated.

Therapist: Ted, let's consider how you can use the problem-solving approach to locate which resources you might need to ask someone out on a date. This time, let's assume you want to ask out a woman from your recreation group. You've talked with her several times now in the past two weeks, but have never asked her out. What's your immediate goal in this situation?

Ted: To ask the woman out.

Therapist: And how will that help you meet your long-term goals?

Ted: It could be a chance to form a closer relationship, which is something I've wanted for a long time.

Therapist: Right. What might you need to ask this woman out?

Ted: Well, I have to choose an activity to do with her, and a time and place to meet. I might also need some money. And I have to decide when to ask her for the date.

Therapist: Very good. Let's start with choosing an activity to do on the date. Can you name some of the things you could do on a date?

Ted: Uh, we could go to the movie or out to dinner, or we could just take a walk somewhere.

Therapist: Let's start with the first possibility. If you were to ask this woman out on a date to the movies and she accepted, tell me as many positive things as you can think of that go along with choosing the movies.

Ted: Well, I like to see the movies, and it's convenient—you can always find some movie to agree on seeing.

Therapist: Can you think of any other advantages?

Ted: You can do it almost any time, so scheduling isn't a problem.

Therapist: Good. How about disadvantages to going to the movies?

Ted: Well, I'd have to shell out money for two tickets, so it would cost me something.

Therapist:—Can you think of any others?

Ted: No.

Therapist: How about you, Karen?

Karen: You can't talk to the person you're with in the movies. That could be a drawback.

Therapist: Good point, Karen!

Therapist: Well, do the advantages outweigh the disadvantages when selecting the movies as an activity?

Ted: I think so. I like the movies, and who doesn't?

Therapist: Okay, then let's practice asking this woman to the movies.

Each time a patient solves resource problems, a number of alternative solutions emerge and can be evaluated. Roleplaying can assure competent implementation of the desired option. In the preceding example, alternative solutions identified by Ted included asking the woman out to dinner or for a walk. If patients have difficulty generating more than one alternative solution, they are asked leading questions to help them identify additional solutions. Patients proceed to apply the problem-solving method to obtain the full array of resources required to use the skills involved in "Making Friends" or "Going on a Date." Examples of resources required are *people* to approach, *places and activities* for spending time with friends, *money, phone,* and *transportation.*

After considering the *resources* necessary to implement a skill, potential *problems and obstacles* to successful attainment of the goal are anticipated, and the same problem-solving approach is used to determine alternative strategies for achieving the goal. As with resource management problems, by the time the last skill area has been reached, 'Going on a Date," the group members are familiar with solving potential outcome problems.

We join our module again after Ted has finished roleplaying asking his woman acquaintance to the movies. In this learning activity, "Solving Outcome Problems," a number of potential obstacles in the patient's pathway to a date are identified by the therapist in advance. Then, potential obstacles or problems anticipated when implementing the dating skills are solved, one at a time, using the same sequence of problem-solving steps: identifying the problem, generating solutions, evaluating solutions, choosing a solution, and implementing it.

Therapist: Ted, I thought you did a real good job of asking for a date in that roleplay. I'd now like you to practice overcoming some obstacles that can crop up when you ask someone out on a date. Karen is going to play Susan, the person who you've just asked out for a date, and I'm going to tell her to present a barricade you could run into in this situation. First, you should try to use your skills as best you can. Second, when you encounter the obstacles I'd like you to employ the problem-solving skills that you've been practicing since the beginning of this group. Do you have any questions?

Ted: No.

     (Therapist takes Karen aside and instructs her to respond to Ted's request for a date with "I don't think so." Then, if Ted tries to figure out why, she should indicate that she doesn't like going to movies and should react favorably to another suggested activity. They return to the group and Karen takes a seat near Ted for the roleplay.)

Therapist: All right. Let's start the roleplay.

Ted: (Turning to face Karen) Hi, Susan, how's it going?

Karen: Okay, how about yourself?

Ted: Can't complain. I was wondering, Susan, if you might want to go to the movies with me tonight?

Karen: No, I don't think so (diffidently).

Therapist: (Stops the roleplaying.) Ted, what's the problem here?

Ted: Trying to get a date!

Therapist: Right, but what's the specific problem you've encountered trying to get the date?

Ted: She turned me down.

Therapist: Right. Now let's use the problem-solving approach. Do you need any money to solve this problem?

Ted: I don't think so, except to have money for the date, and I've already planned for that.

Therapist: Good. How about the skills to solve this problem. Do you think you have the skills to solve this problem?

Ted: I think so. I've been practicing talking with women a lot, and I think I'm better at it.

Therapist: How about people, do you need any people to solve this problem?

Ted: I need Susan, but no one else. But if she keeps turning me down, then I might try someone else.

Therapist: That's a good point, you can always ask someone else out if it doesn't work out with Susan. But to try getting a date with Susan, you don't need anyone else.

Ted: Right.

Therapist: Well, what could you do to try and solve the problem?

Ted: I could ask her out tomorrow night instead of tonight. Maybe the time isn't good.

Therapist: If you ask her out tomorrow night instead of tonight would you achieve your goal?

Ted: Maybe, it's hard to tell.

Therapist: What are the advantages of asking her out tomorrow night?

Ted: I might find out if she had a problem with the time.

Therapist: Any disadvantages to asking her out tomorrow night?

Ted: Maybe she just doesn't like going to the movies.

Therapist: Good. Can you think of another alternative solution for how you might deal with this problem?

Ted: I could ask her if she's busy. That would leave things kind of open.

Therapist: Would that solution solve the problem?

Ted: It might.

Therapist: What are the advantages to that solution?

Ted: Well, I would find out if she didn't want to go because she was busy or because she didn't like movies.

Therapist: What are the disadvantages you can think of?

Ted: I might find out that she doesn't like *me*.

Therapist: Or that she doesn't want to go out with you?

Ted: Yeah. But I suppose it's better knowing than not knowing.

Therapist: At least you would know where you stand. Which of these two alternative solutions is better: asking her out tomorrow night or asking if she's busy?

Ted: I think it's better to ask if she's busy tonight. I would find out more about why she can't go tonight.

Therapist: Good. Let's continue with this roleplay and evaluate this alternative solution . . .

This process of solving outcome problems is repeated with each patient with a number of potential obstacles. For example, other obstacles that could be problem solved for the "Going on a Date" skill area include the other person refusing all requests for a date or the other person not showing up at the prearranged time for the date. A list of different outcome problems that can be used in this learning activity is presented in Table 4-3. Naturally, the specific types of problems that a patient might encounter depend on the individual's affluence, social networks and social support, and living arrangements. Therefore, specific resource management problems and outcome problems for training need to be constructed to meet the individual needs of the patients participating in the group.

We follow up our group of patients one last time at the end of their participation in the Friendship and Dating Skills module. Ted was successful in going on a date with Susan, and they have gone out two more times since then. In addition to reporting his positive experiences in going out on some dates, Ted's tendency to become easily frustrated and angry was improved by anticipating outcome problems in the different

Table 4-3. Examples of Obstacles or Outcome Problems in the "Going on a Date" Skill Area

- The person you are interested in does not want to go on a date.
- The person you want to date is interested in going on a date but has scheduling problems or does not like the activity you suggested.
- Your prospective date does not show up at the agreed-upon time.
- Your date claims to feel ill while in the midst of the date.
- Your date suddenly decides that a different activity than the one planned would be desirable.
- Your date appears bored and indifferent.
- Your date comes on unexpectedly strong with interest and affection.

skill areas. This enabled him to have a planned course of action when others thwarted him from achieving his goals.

Karen also reported going out on several dates and was pleased that her anxiety while conversing with men decreased even more. As Karen has become more comfortable interacting with men, she has been asked out on more dates, and needed to practice refusing dates assertively with men in whom she was not interested.

Carol went out on one date and Allen did not go out on any, but both showed gains in their ability to establish friendships. Allen has made a friend at his day treatment program, and they sometimes get together over weekends to listen to music. Allen is still not very active socially, but he reports more comfort in his interaction and appears less bored and detached during conversations than before. Carol has also established the beginnings of a friendship and has been spending more time with her friends and less time with her family. In sum, the module has helped its members to deepen their interpersonal relationships with others.

SUMMARY

Psychiatric patients frequently complain about the lack of social support, including companionship and friendly relationships with others. Even when patients have adequate social and independent living skills, their ability to start and maintain new relationships often remains impaired. Poor social and sexual adjustment before the onset of illness remains a very potent predictor of poor adjustment later. A key to understanding the importance of this set of skills is the high level of motivation shown by patients as they get involved in learning friendship and dating skills.

A module for training affiliative skills is designed to teach patients several related skills areas in sequence. The very same social skills training techniques described in the last chapter are used to teach friendship and dating skills. Since patients often experience common kinds of problems with handling intimacy, the problem-solving method used in social skills is an important tool for the patient to possess. In learning how to make friends, patients are taught to define the problems and challenges they face, generate alternative solutions, evaluate the alternatives, select the best one, and use it effectively.

Problems encountered in friendship and dating situations are sorted into two types: resource management and outcome. Resources are the materials and logistics a person needs for successful dating, including money, telephone, clothes, and transportation. Outcome problems are the often unanticipated and frustrating obstacles encountered when attempting to use new dating skills such as rejection of an invitation for a date. The problem-solving approach is learned for managing resource and outcome problems.

The Friendship and Dating Skills module is best taught in groups of four to twelve patients, but the sessions should meet three times a week for 90 minutes over two to four months. Patients should be competent in basic conversational and self-care skills to increase their chances of success. They should be able to engage in roleplaying since nine standard "scenes" are used to assess initial skill levels.

Four skills areas are taught in order: initiating conversations with strangers, recognizing and expressing emotions, making friends, and going on a date. Roleplay activities for each of these areas are used and the module focuses on solving the resource and outcome problems that patients are likely to encounter. The module contains assessment scenarios, component social skills for the four skill areas, and examples of obstacles or outcome problems for the "Going on a Date" skill area.

Chapter 5
Overcoming Resistance to Social Skills Training

Social skills trainers should assume that all patients are always doing the very best they can, given their psychobiological endowment, previous learning experiences, and current environmental resources. Resistance to change is not so much willful negativism or a temporary block within the patient to be breached, but rather exists for good reasons that must be understood and grappled with. By crafting the learning process and the helping relationship, the therapist or trainer can build motivation and a desire to participate in social skills training for even the most reluctant and low-functioning patients. This chapter will provide ideas and a framework for helping patients to move forward with their learning and application of social skills.

The best "cure" for resistance to social skills training is to prevent its occurrence in the first place. Preventing or minimizing resistance entails developing rapport and a solid therapeutic alliance from the very start—even before a patient attends his or her first assessment or training session. For example, one of the most critical determinants of patients' participation and attendance in social skills training is the way in which the referral or invitation to join the group is made. The following points can be useful guidelines when patients are being readied to join a group.

- Have the patient's primary therapist or responsible psychiatrist provide an affirmative rationale and orientation for joining the social skills training group. This may require some consultation between the leader(s) of the group and the referring professional.
- The patient's primary therapist or responsible psychiatrist should, if possible, come with the patient for the first skills training session, sit in, and lend support to the assessment and training efforts related to the new patient.

- Provide the patient, in advance, with a brochure or written information—pegged at a layperson's level of comprehension—that communicates the rationale for the training and builds favorable, yet realistic, expectations for what transpires in the group.

A sample orientation brochure is reprinted in Appendix A to this guidebook. We encourage you to photocopy this brochure, or design and print one of your own that better fits your clinical setting and group format, and distribute them to patients prior to their attending an initial training session. From the appended orientation brochure you can see how the patient's expectation for a positive experience and outcome are raised, even while predicting some of the discomforts that require adaptation. The patient is informed about the role of the therapist as well as the patient, including modeling and homework assignments. The patient is told what will happen, when, and why. Preparing the patient for specific elements of the training or therapy procedure cannot be done only once at the start of treatment, but repeatedly presented as skills training proceeds.

EFFECTIVE PLANNING
PREEMPTS RESISTANCE

There is challenge in forming an effective therapeutic relationship with a psychiatric patient—especially with patients lacking in insight and in whom cognitive deficits, medication side effects, and negativism are inherent in the nature of their very disorder. Engaging a patient in a structured program of skills training requires considerable planning as well as therapeutic skill, enthusiasm, and persistence. Several steps can be followed in planning the social skills training program that will promote a working alliance subsequently with patients:

- Assess the needs of the patients.
- Clearly formulate the training objectives and build favorable expectations.
- Undercut efforts to "defeat" the therapist or the program or skills training.
- Plan the specific structure of the training, including the use of motivational aids and prompts.

Assess the Needs of the Patients

Without having a clear picture of the needs and social network of the patients you wish to treat, your training program may be hit or miss. For example, if the patients are young adults with schizophrenia who are living at home with relatives, it would be important to include the relatives in some part of the training. This will make allies of the relatives who can become supporters (rather than saboteurs) of the training program. Assessment interviews can be conducted with the relatives—preferably in their homes—as well as with the patient, exploring his or her individual strengths and weaknesses as well as their family culture, expectations, emotional climate, and transactions. If the family is involved in the therapeutic process from the start (or even better at the time of the patient's hospitalization or intake into the clinic), the family members' support and participation with the patient in skills training will be more continuous. There are several ways to accomplish this as indicated in the following vignettes.

Karen's mother, with whom she lives, was invited to participate in occasional social skills training sessions. This was especially helpful for facilitating Karen's goals because the mother learned how to give Karen praise and encouragement for pursuing more social initiative and independence.

Ted, who was estranged from his parents, introduced the operator and manager of his board-and-care home to the trainer. The trainer then worked out an agreement that Ted's homework assignments would be shared with the operator and manager who would make opportunities available for Ted to complete the assignments. Once, when Ted was aiming to join a social club sponsored by a church, his home manager provided transportation to the church, which was located across town.

Carol's parents were invited to attend a family education group and to meet monthly with Carol and the social skills trainer to review her progress and plan ways to facilitate her achieving greater independence. At one meeting, they agreed to purchase a car for her transportation needs if she was successful in being accepted into a vocational rehabilitation program.

In other cases, the needs of the patients for social skills training may become salient only after more pressing needs are first taken care of. For example, patients at risk for losing their disability pensions, or who are facing termination from their primary therapist or psychiatrist, or who are homeless will require intervention to deal with these more pressing needs prior to engaging in a course of social skills training.

It is also incumbent upon the therapist to assist the patient in formulating the reasons for coming to a mental health professional *now*. Future resistance to inappropriately chosen goals and techniques can be obviated by employing a "customer" approach with the patient. In doing this, the therapist helps the patient articulate poorly understood needs and wishes and actively pursues the patient's hopes, fears, and desires for change and for the treatment experience itself.

Set Training Objectives and Build Favorable Expectations

Once the needs of the patients are identified, it is much easier to proceed to plan the objectives of the training program and to build favorable expectations for the training. For example, persons may be inadequate in social relationships, not because of deficits in social skills, but because of unrealistically underestimating their skills and consequently avoiding social situations. This is very frequent in patients with anxiety and affective disorders, with their symptoms leading to a vicious cycle of low self-esteem, loss of confidence in social situations, avoidance of social contacts, failure to use their repertoire of social skills, more loss of self-esteem, and so on. In this situation, the objectives of training would center on providing patients with a clear rationale for skills training. The rationale should include restructuring social expectations, being willing to experience awkwardness in social situations, entering relatively simple situations initially to gain confidence, and accepting the training process as a means of obtaining extra motivation to get back on track with skills already possessed, but rusty.

Building favorable expectations may have to include descriptions and education on how the patient's psychiatric illness may be helped by something as unfamiliar as skills training. Describe the biopsychosocial model of disease and to the "stress-vulnerability-coping-competence" framework for understanding serious mental disorders (See p. 231 of Annotated Bibliography), elucidating the ways in which skills result in improved coping and competence that can displace or buffer intrusive psychopathology. Information about symptoms and the ways in which psychotropic medication and skills training mutually facilitate each other's therapeutic effects in countering symptoms can also be helpful in convincing a patient to join a skills training group.

Joe, a 39-year-old lawyer with a major depression, agreed to participate in social skills training only after it was explained that antidepressant medication could improve his insomnia, loss of interests, and mood but that only social skills training could equip him with the ability to overcome his problems in communicating his affection to and need for reciprocity from his wife—which were triggers in his depression and would continue to keep him vulnerable to future depressive episodes.

It is well-accepted and empirically documented that adequate orientation to the particular treatment being offered will promote favorable expectations and better outcome for the patient. In social skills training, realistic expectations are easier to inculcate by virtue of the concrete, down-to-earth, and direct nature of the training methods. Rationales are particularly important for patients with chronic problems where confusion about the disorder has been fed by multiple and frustrating experiences with therapists of differing persuasions. Behavioral practitioners are well versed in rationales that can help to clear up confusion in patients suffering from agoraphobia; for example, explaining how environmental over-stimulation of a vulnerable autonomic nervous system can produce recognizable symptoms and how escape from or avoidance of feared situations reinforces the phobia.

TRAINING DIFFICULT AND REFRACTORY PATIENTS

In Chapter 3, we presented an example of a social skills training session with a patient whose schizophrenia was in reasonably good remission. Carol's skills were in evidence even before her illness began and were readily mobilized by the structure and motivational features of the training steps. While she had obvious skills deficits and social anxieties, she was an eager learner and was no management problem in the training group.

"But anyone can do this kind of treatment with patients like that," we hear you saying, "I need help with some of the tough ones, the ones like Ted or Allen." But of course. And you've come to the right place in the book. Let's tune in on a later part of the same session described in Chapter 3, as the therapist begins working with Ted.

Therapist: All right, Ted. It's your turn. You were going to practice giving constructive criticism today. Do you have any situation in particular that you'd like to practice?

Ted: Naw. It's dumb. I don't want to anymore. I'm doin' okay now. I don't have to give criticism. I just tell 'em, and they straighten up.

Therapist: Well, sometimes things don't turn out so well, right?

Ted: Yeah, well, if people would leave me alone, things would be better. When things don't go so well, I just split. I don't even have to stay here and play these silly games.

Therapist: It sounds as if you did well on your assignment. I know how difficult that was for you. And you were very helpful to Carol by taking the role of "bus driver." Although practicing your own skills and goals isn't easy, why don't you show us how you gave the compliment to Mr. Houk, the supervisor at your job. I know he's not your favorite person.

Ted: No doubt. He's a real jerk sometimes. He gets mad too easy. He shouldn't be allowed to be in charge. He doesn't even like half of us who work there.

Therapist: Who reminds you of Mr. Houk, Ted? Who could do a good job playing him?

Ted: I dunno. I don't want to do this today. Just skip me, okay?

Therapist: I understand how you feel, Ted. Let's just do a brief scene, to see how you did. You know we try to have everyone practice something every session, even if it's short.

Ted: All right. But it better be quick. I'm gettin' hungry too. When can we go for lunch?

Therapist: Not too much longer, Ted. I'm pleased that you'll show how you handled the assignment. Besides, doing things when you don't feel like it is important. Well, let's get going. Who could be Mr. Houk, Ted?

Ted: That new guy, Mark. He's big, like Houk.

Therapist: Tell us how you started the conversation, and how he reacted.

Ted: I did what we practiced last time. I went up to him when he wasn't real busy, when all the jobs were done. He was reading the newspaper at his desk. He kind of ignores you at first. Makes you feel kind of stupid.

Therapist: OK. Mark, you sit here and pretend to read the paper. Show us how it went, Ted.

(Mark sits and pretends to read the paper. Ted approaches from the side. The therapist moves to where he can watch Ted's face.)

Ted: (Softly) Uh, Mr. Houk. (Mark doesn't respond. Ted repeats, a little louder.) Mr. Houk.

Mark: (Still reading) What?

Ted: Nothing. I just wanted to tell you that I appreciate your getting that catering truck to come over to the shop for our coffee and lunch breaks. A lot of companies don't let you do that. It makes it more like home.

Mark: (Still reading) OK. But be sure you don't take advantage and use more than the time you're given.

Ted: Right. We'll keep an eye on the clock.

Therapist: Cut right here. Good. What good things did you notice about Ted's performance, Karen?

Karen: He spoke up. He got his supervisor's attention, and he got right to the point. He didn't get too close, though.

Therapist: Yes. He got within four or five feet. He didn't make Mr. Houk uncomfortable. Allen, what did you notice?

Allen: Eye contact.

Therapist: What about eye contact?

Allen: He looked at him when he talked.

Therapist: Good, Allen. He did. He did very well. Ted, while we're at it, why don't you try to bring up the subject of using a radio at work for background music.

Ted: OK. I guess I could try. But it's kind of tough.

Therapist: Yes, it is. It's always hard to try to get someone to talk about changing rules. Why don't you and Mark pick it up where you left off?

Mark: (To Ted) By the way, Ted, keep that ghetto blaster of yours off after lunch break. You know the rules.

Ted: Just a second. I don't think that's fair. Why can't we listen to music while we're working? (Now Ted is waving his arms around, gesturing broadly—and wildly.)

Mark: Well, that's one of the rules.

Ted: Who made that rule up? Nobody asked ME!

Mark: Now, just cool down. I made that rule when we had some workers here who didn't want to have to listen to that stuff all day.

Ted: I'll tell you what you can do . . .

Therapist: Cut! Carol, what are some of the things that Ted did right?

Carol: Well, he got pretty mad . . .

Therapist: Yes, but focus on some of the things he did right before he got mad.

Carol: Uh . . . (thinks awhile) . . . I don't know. He did have good eye contact, and he still didn't get in too close. He told him what he thought of the rule.

Therapist: True, he kept his distance and got right to the point. What could he have done to improve?

Carol: Not get so mad. He probably would get Mr. Houk mad too, if he did that.

Ted: Yeah, yeah. I know.

Therapist: That's right. Good! Thank you, Carol. Let's look at how you handled that situation. Ted, what did Mr. Houk say to you?

Ted: He said: "Turn that damn radio off after lunch." He said it was just his rule, and that's what got me upset. I don't like it when people act like dictators.

Therapist: That's close to what he said, Ted. What did he say exactly? Anyone?

Karen: He said something like "Keep that ghetto blaster off after lunch. You know the rules." He didn't say it angry.

Therapist: Good observation, Karen. Ted, what do you think Mr. Houk was feeling during that exchange?

Ted: Do we have to go through this? I know I screwed up. I guess he was getting mad. He probably wasn't at first, but later he was getting mad.

Therapist: What was it that would have made him mad?

Ted: I got up in his face. I yelled at him. But he deserved it. I don't think he likes me.

Therapist: What were your short-term goals in that situation?

Ted: I think, uh. . . . Yeah, to discuss the rule against playing the radio and to get him to change his stupid rule.

Therapist: And the long-term goals?

Ted: You mean, like later?

Therapist: What was it that you wanted to happen after you had this conversation with Mr. Houk?

Ted: Oh. I guess to enjoy a nicer work environment and to have him treat us like adults.

Therapist: Right! What about having a better future working relationship with Houk? Do you think you would have achieved that by talking the way you did?

Ted: Hell, no. I'd have probably gotten thrown out.

Therapist: What could you have done differently that would have helped reach your goals?

Ted: I know, I know. You don't have to tell me. Keep my cool. Keep my voice down. Don't wave my arms around. Talk nice.

Therapist: And what could you have said to get your point across—I mean, specifically and effectively?

Ted: Uh, something like, "Could we talk about changing that no music rule?" or "Maybe if we all agree to keep the volume turned way down, could we have some more time to listen to music while we're working?"

Therapist: Good, Ted. I'm impressed. You have some good ideas on how to handle that situation better. Let's get some more ideas from others in the group and have someone else show us how they might do it.

As you can see from this exchange, dealing with the patient who has more socially maladaptive excesses than deficits can be a lot of work.

Here, the therapist was faced with a person who suddenly became resistive. It is a challenge to cajole, humor, or otherwise motivate such a person into doing something in a session and to not allow him or her to avoid practice. Dropping back to demonstrating the successful assignment was a good ploy to use with Ted, and when the therapist took a chance of pressing on, Ted went along with the suggestion and actually went on to complete the practice originally planned.

Flexibility and Patience Yields Progress

As with any other situation where you are trying to motivate a patient into doing something that he or she doesn't want to do, never let the situation escalate into a power struggle. Be flexible, but be clever. Maintain the normal expectation of every patient performing at every session, but present alternatives rather than just restate the rule. Keep your options open, and be a moving target. Never let the exchange deteriorate to the "You will! . . . I won't!" stage. Can you imagine what would have happened if the therapist had tried to bully Ted into performing? Not only would the therapist have presented an inappropriate model to the rest of the group, but he would have stood an excellent chance of losing Ted entirely, not to mention provoking an aggressive incident!

With Ted, the problem-solving portion of the session is very important. His receiving and processing skills need a good deal of work. It is obvious that he has certain expectations about interactions with other people and that he distorts what they say or do to fulfill those expectations. He fully expected Mr. Houk to become angry, and through his aggressive behavior, managed to provoke him. Ted's lack of problem-solving skills renders him unable to identify appropriate responses during a conflict situation. When other people disagree with him or criticize him, he can't think of what to say, and he begins to feel anxious and trapped. Often, people who feel trapped exaggerate others' intentions or feelings and have difficulty thinking of solutions to a problem. As a consequence, they become aggressive and strike out at those around them. While aggressive behavior releases stress and tension temporarily, such relief is illusory because it comes at the cost of thwarting the achievement of short- and long-term goals.

Getting Ted to break that chain of events is a real key to having him become socially effective and having a more stable life. Notice that interpreting Ted's social distortions or giving him insight into them was bypassed in favor of directly teaching him to perceive correctly his interpersonal partner's feelings and attitudes. Insight will come later as a natural consequence of Ted's improved relationships.

Occasionally you will encounter a new patient who is resistant to behavioral rehearsal, despite your attempts to engage him or her by using the strategies previously described. Some of these patients are "therapist killers" who take pride in the number of different therapists who have failed to "cure" them. Other times, patients are either extremely dubious that the methods will work for them or are actively suspicious or paranoid about roleplaying in the group. When it is clear to you that your best efforts will not succeed in getting a patient to roleplay, then you need to head off a confrontation by giving the patient permission not to roleplay at this time, while setting the expectation that he or she will roleplay in a future session.

Once patients have begun to attend the social skills training group and are able to observe other patients roleplaying and improving their skills through behavioral rehearsal, their resistance begins to break down as they see others benefiting from the practice. Furthermore, group process and the newly formed relationships with others in the group serve as social support to patients, encouraging them to participate and cheering them on as they improve. Knowing when to refrain from trying to persuade patients further to roleplay is critical for maintaining a therapeutic relationship with them and ultimately engaging their cooperation in social skills training. Patience, flexibility, and understanding on the part of the therapist can go a long way toward motivating resistant patients to participate in behavioral rehearsal.

With Allen, the challenge is very different. He could be described as a social isolate. He is much less exciting to work with than is Ted, or even Carol, and the task is to increase the amount and intensity of his social interactions. At the moment, both the amount and intensity are practically nonexistent, especially outside of his limited daily routine. It is more exhausting having Allen in the group than Ted. With severely impaired and disabled patients, it is almost as if one of the laws of physics has been repealed: You can get Allen moving by pushing hard, but when you stop, he stops. Inertia is always there, but not momentum. With some patients who fit this description, learning basic and elementary conversation skills may be a prerequisite "course" before going on to higher-level social skills training. The same principles are used in basic conversation skills, but the skills practiced are the building blocks of social interaction: eye contact; approaching a conversational partner; audible speech; beginning, maintaining, and ending conversations. (A special "module" as well as a syllabus for professionals wishing to teach basic conversational skills are available from the UCLA Clinical Research Center by writing to the first author of this guidebook.)

Allen is a marginal candidate for basic conversation skills training. Let's look at how the therapist conducts a practice session with Allen.

Remember, voice loudness and eye contact were targeted for practice when the assignments were reviewed.

Therapist: Allen, let's work on speaking louder and looking at the person you're talking to. Would you come over here? Who would you like to practice having a conversation with today?

Allen: (He doesn't move or look up.) Mmaak.

Therapist: Will you repeat that, Allen? I thought you said "Mark."

Allen: Mark.

Therapist: Well, Mark is new here, and we usually let a new person introduce himself on the first day, and then just observe. Have you been introduced to Mark yet?

Allen: No.

Therapist: Well, if Mark is willing, let's use this session as a way to practice meeting someone new and starting a brief conversation. Mark, is that all right with you? Will you help out in this scene? You just have to be yourself.

Mark: I think so. All right.

Therapist: Let's keep this very simple. Allen, I want you to introduce yourself to Mark. Just pretend you don't already know his name. Get him to tell you his name, and find out where he lives. Shake his hand. Let's say this room is just outside the building here. You've noticed that Mark is a new person in the group, and you want to get acquainted. The first step in getting to meet someone new is what, Allen? Remember, we practiced this first step last week.

Allen: You mean to introduce yourself?

Therapist: Correct! So, you will introduce yourself. Mark would you come over here?

(The therapist again moves to where she can see Allen's face. She guides Allen to a spot about six or seven feet away from Mark.)

Therapist: (Allen moves forward exactly two feet, tentatively holds out his hand, and speaks softly and hurriedly.)

Mark: (Mark looks confused and starts forward to approach Allen. He reaches out for Allen's hand, but as he does, Allen looks away and withdraws his hand.)

Therapist: Let's stop there. Allen, stay right here. What did Allen do that was positive? Carol?

Carol: Well, he started toward Mark, and I think he introduced himself, but I couldn't hear, and he held out his hand for a handshake.

Therapist: Anyone else? Ted?

Ted: I don't know. He stopped at the last minute before Mark could shake his hand, but he had a friendly expression.

Therapist: Yes, Allen's facial expression was very encouraging to Mark. Let's have Ted demonstrate for Allen how to improve his voice volume and speech fluency. Then we'll have Allen practice the same situation again.

(Notice that the therapist finds something in the performance to reward with group approval, even in this limited situation with obvious, gross deficits in Allen's performance in the dry run. At this point, the therapist then uses a model to show Allen how this introduction might be done by someone else. In Allen's case, it is especially important to be certain that he is actually watching the model, even to the point of checking to see that his eyes are open during the model's performance! After the model demonstrates the introduction, the therapist runs Allen through the scene again. This time he has made substantial improvements in all sending skills but voice loudness and eye contact. The therapist now uses prompting to help get him to keep his voice, and eyes, up in conversation.)

Therapist: Allen, I'm going to stand behind Mark this time. When I want you to speak louder, I'll signal, like this (holds his right hand out, palm up and parallel to the floor, moving it up). When I want you to look at Mark, I'll do this (points to his eye). Got it? OK. Go.

Allen: (Approaches Mark and offers his hand) Hi. I'm Allen. (Therapist gestures for more volume.) Who . . . What's your name? (Therapist points to his eyes, Allen looks more directly at Mark.)

Mark: Mark. (Shakes his hand. Allen withdraws his quickly, looks down. Therapist points vigorously at his own eyes, and Allen takes the cue again, looking in the general direction of Mark.) Have you been coming here long? This is my first session. What's it like?

Allen: No, not long. It's not too bad. (Therapist gestures for more volume.) Where do you live?

Mark: Over on Sixth Street. Where do you live?

Allen: (His gaze begins to drift, and the therapist points rapidly to his eyes.) Near the park. On Catalpa Street. Take the bus.

Mark: No, I uh . . . do you mean, "Do I take the bus?" or do you? I get dropped off here. My brother drives me.

Allen: I get the 44 bus. Costs fifty cents.

Therapist: Cut it there! Very nice, Allen. Karen, what did Allen do well in that scene?

Karen: He was much better. I could hear him, and he looked at him more. And he gave Mark some "free" information about riding the bus. He did better.

The therapist reinforces the positive feedback given by the other group members highlighting Allen's distinct improvement over his first performance. Karen picked up on the fact that Allen had actually brought up a new subject on his own (the fact that he rides the bus, the "free" information she mentioned). This is one of the basic skills that patients learn in conversation training. Mark could then react to the "free" information and keep the conversation going.

Therapist: Allen, for an assignment, I want you to begin at least two conversations with your sister Jane or anyone else, and I am writing on the assignment card that I would like them to notice your eye contact and voice loudness. Here's your assignment card.

Treatment Tool Kit

In the examples of behavioral rehearsal given in this chapter, we have presented some of the most common types of problem behaviors you might encounter. While every patient is unique, we have developed some useful exercises for problems seen frequently in patients with major mental illness. This list is not exhaustive, but it represents the most frequently used techniques. We are certain that you will be able to invent some of your own. The exercises that follow serve an energizing purpose as well, since they involve exaggerated action and more activity from those involved.

1. "Louder!" For patients like Allen who mumble or speak very softly, this technique gives them practice in speaking up. If it is a strain to hear a person speaking, it is also not very rewarding to carry on that exchange. Maintaining proper voice volume is a basic step in the shaping of conversational and assertiveness skills and other, more complex social and emotional behaviors.

Having the patient and the person with whom he or she is supposed to converse stand far apart (perhaps 10 to 20 feet) and hold their conversation *as if* they were standing together makes it necessary for them to speak very loudly. If the distances are a problem in your setting, have one party stand outside the room and converse. The therapist prompts the patient during this strange conversation, encouraging him or her to raise and maintain voice volume. When the patient can be heard clearly, a great deal of approval should be shown by all present.

Rather than use two patients in this situation, you might find it more efficient to be the "interpersonal target" for the patient. Here, you can instruct the patient that you will give him or her a signal to speak louder and another signal when the volume is satisfactory.

2. "How Low Can You Go?" Voice tone is extremely important in conveying information and feeling. The same message can evoke entirely

different responses in the listener if the tone of voice is pleasant or if it's strained. Four exercises can help teach control of tone:

- To find your optimum pitch, repeat the sentence "I don't think it's going to rain" while lowering your voice a half tone at each repetition. When it becomes uncomfortable, raise your voice one full tone. This should be close to your optimum tone.
- Relaxing the throat muscles during speech is necessary for many patients. Pressing the tongue against the roof of the mouth and then relaxing it several times is one approach to easing the tension. Relaxing and contracting the jaw muscles and yawning and sighing are two other exercises that will achieve the same effect.
- Deep breathing exercises, which involve deep breathing, holding the breath, and then releasing it, are commonly found in progressive relaxation methods and can relax the chest muscles.
- Energizing the voice can be achieved by speaking with the chest up and out, the diaphragm pulled in and up toward the spine.

3. "The Silent Movie." For those who speak moving only their lips, devoid of facial expression or gestures, the Silent Movie is just the ticket. The therapist tells the patient to express an emotion (e.g., joy, sorrow, annoyance) to another person. The object of the exercise is to express the emotion using only facial expression, hand gestures, and body posture. As in the old silent movies themselves, the gestures and expressions must be exaggerated if the message is to be conveyed. Common situations can be used: Express annoyance to a relative or friend, show appreciation to someone who has done you a favor, show pleasure at being asked to go on an outing.

4. "Positive Statements." This is an extremely useful procedure in which a person is told to carry out a conversation on a particular subject without using any negative, derogatory, or depressing statements. If this sounds too much like Pollyanna, remember that there are people we converse with who see the dark side of any topic. Without knowing why, we find ourselves becoming depressed, as well, and avoiding them. To sensitize such patients and to teach them how to break the cycle of gloom, positive statements can be employed. Set a time limit for the conversation, say, one or two minutes, and you may be surprised at how difficult it is for some people to go for that long without bringing up something negative. For them, it's harder than it sounds!

5. "Broken Record." This is one of the most effective and valuable tools in the box. For patients and nonpatients alike, it provides them

with a device for accomplishing their goals quickly. It is also unnerving to carry out at first! The basic principle that must be learned is that when faced with a difficult person who is insistent (for example) that you do something you do not want to do, you do not have to come up with new and improved reasons for not going along with the repeated nagging and cajoling of the other person. The key task is to decide on your message ("I don't want to go tonight") and stick to it. Reasons are not necessary. Responses take the form of "I don't want to go." "I really don't want to go." "No, I don't feel like it." "I don't want to go." Once this pattern of responses is set up, it becomes very difficult for the aggressor to get through. This technique can give patients a new sense of control over relationships. And, just as important, it can be used to express a positive desire as well.

6. "Fogging." Closely related to Broken Record, Fogging can be described as the iron will in Teddy Bear's clothing. Simply reflecting the other person's request and adding ". . . but I'm sorry, I can't do that," conveys two messages. The first is that the patient has heard and understands how important the request is to the other person, and the second states mild regret that the patient simply does not desire to go along with the request. Done in the most solicitous, perhaps even unctuous tones, Fogging is effective at keeping hurt feelings down to a mild bruise. For example, when pressure is placed on a person to join an activity, Fogging could be stating, "I know you really want me to go, but I can't tonight." Repeated and restated, it becomes more and more like a Broken Record.

Notice that no explanations or heavy-duty apologies are permitted. A third message is sent in this way: "I can make my mind up about things without having to explain them or apologize. I will do things when I feel like it. Back off!"

7. "Psst! Hey, Buddy, C'mere." It is also unpleasant to converse with those who are not very fluent in their speech. Many patients have words that they want to say, but have trouble saying them. Long pauses, meaningless "filler" sounds, and a lack of energy and continuity make conversing a chore for the listener. By contrast, the skills needed to carry out a sales pitch require fluency above all else. Having the patient convince you or another person to purchase something is a useful vehicle for this. By placing a time limit of one or two minutes on this exercise, also called "Sell me something," and counting the filler sounds, such as "Uh" and "Y'know" and long pauses, the barriers to fluency can be identified and eliminated. The first time through, the patient may have difficulty, but by the second or third rehearsal, he or she should show improvement. The idea is not to make salespersons out of the patients, but to give them a concrete exercise in which they can increase their fluency while talking to other people.

8. "Executive Session." Used heavily with couples and others who are in danger of becoming intimate enemies, the Executive Session slows down communication and concentrates attention on understanding the messages being sent by both parties. The first person to speak states a point of view, either a want or need, and waits until the second party has restated that message in such a manner that the first party agrees that the message has been received and processed properly. At that point, the second party gets to speak. If it sounds strange here, it sounds even stranger the first time you hear it done. But the intent is to drain off the emotional charge in a difficult situation and to have the players concentrate on the content of the message the other person is sending. For example,

Wife: You never pick up after yourself. You must think I'm some kind of slave. When I have to turn your dirty socks right side out, I feel angry and upset! You wouldn't treat your mother like that!

Husband: I hear you saying that you want me to stop dropping my clothes on the floor and that it makes you angry when I leave them around.

Wife: That's right.

And then the husband gets to state his point of view, and the wife has to reflect back what her husband has said, checking with him regarding the accuracy of her understanding of his intent *before* she goes on to express her next point. Besides slowing down emotionally charged discussions and arguments, the Executive Session provides the people involved with a way to de-escalate tension and hostility and remain in a constructive problem-solving mode.

Warm-up Exercises

Pacing a training session is as important as its structure, because there is so much to do with each patient that you have to keep moving so as not to run out of time or risk losing your audience. Sometimes, it seems that no matter how dynamic you try to be, the group just doesn't respond. You find yourself having to drag every response from the group members, and it seems as if you are the only one really awake and interested in what's happening. Sound familiar? What follows is a bag of tricks that we have found useful to "jump start" a sluggish group. They are general-use situations that are familiar to everyone and may be used at any point in the session. Some therapists like to end a session by using these "warm-up exercises" or "stock" scenes because they are fun to do and can be spontaneous aids to easing into the more serious training process. For the alert therapist, they can be more than just entertainment. By watching patients go through these scenes, it is often possible to spot deficits or excesses in skills that might otherwise have gone unnoticed. This list is by no means exhaustive, and you will naturally find others that will work just as well.

1. "Line Jumpers." Group members form a line waiting to buy tickets at a box office. Some in the front of the line invite some friends to join them. How do those in line react? How good is the social judgment of those involved? How accurately do the aggrieved patrons in line assess the situation? How big and how many are the line jumpers for instance! In the real world, discretion is sometimes best, but certainly not always!

2. "Ptomaine Palace." This is a restaurant scene in which a variety of unpleasant things may happen. The order is wrong; the meat is "off"; the plates/flatware are not clean; there's a fly in my soup; the waiter/waitress hasn't taken our order yet; the bill is wrong (in the restaurant's favor); there was a piece of chocolate cream pie left on my chair, and I sat in it (real situation!); and the rest of the litany of woes that can beset the casual gourmet out on the town. Resist, however, the approach taken by Jack Nicholson in the classic restaurant scene in the movie *Five Easy Pieces*. He can get away with grossly insulting a waitress and trashing a restaurant in a movie. We are trying to teach social skills, not social assault. Neither we nor our patients can do the same without risking our safety and freedom!

3. "Cash, Please." A person is returning that wonderfully colorful shirt, gift courtesy of Uncle Mel, to the department store. You have no sales receipt, and even Mel wasn't exactly sure from which store in the chain he bought it in the first place. Not only do you wish to return it, but you want a cash refund instead of a credit slip.

4. "Mr. Badwrench." The car has been into the shop for the fifth time for the same reason. It still tries to accelerate briskly, but without benefit of you pressing the throttle pedal. The mechanic says something vague about these new computerized engines and tries to tell you that "They all do that." You want it fixed, now, for good.

5. "Bethlehem Blues, or No Room at the Ramada." You arrive tired and rumpled from a long trip, and the clerk at the hotel desk can't seem to find your reservation. Your wife is in an advanced state of freeway fatigue, and your kids in the car could audition for a new version of *Vacation*. Having the clerk make amends by finding you something in this establishment or arranging for a room in another, nearby, motel is the goal here.

6. "Looky Lou." Go to a new car showroom and ask to test drive a car. Tell the salesman that you are not at all sure that you are serious about buying. Try to keep his interest, and get that test drive!

7. "But Officer." Any routine situation in which a person has been stopped by an officer is just fine. Usually, only two people are involved unless the officer has a partner or the person who is stopped has other people in the car. This scene is effective because it provokes real anxiety in many people. It should be realistic and genuinely instructive, since the consequences of poor receiving, processing, and sending skills here can be most unpleasant. We have found it useful to obtain some consultation about what behavior police officers expect when making routine stops, and what it is that annoys or interferes with their duty. Play this "straight," and it may have good consequences for the patients. This includes dealing with officers who may not be as courteous as they could be or who may stop you for reasons you don't agree are valid.

8. "Commercially Available Games." You can purchase games in toy or department stores that evoke active social participation and provide good "warm-ups" for a stolid group of patients. One of these games is called "Pit" (Parker Bros.) and requires members of the group to shout out loud the names of commodities they wish to trade in a game that simulates the Chicago Commodities Exchange. Another one is the "Dating Game," which requires participants to ask questions of each other after rolling the dice and moving their pieces around a game board. As can be seen in Figure 5-1, the conversational turn-taking structure inherent in a game can markedly enhance the level of social interaction in a group, even when the group members suffer from chronic schizophrenia.

In all these scenes, use as many patients and staff as you can. The idea is to get as many people up and doing as possible, so put in all the "extras" you can. This also can make for a very lifelike situation. As an example, when running the "Cash Please" scene, it's really more realistic to have other customers at the counter or cash register vying for the salesperson's attention. An even tougher situation is to have the salesperson waiting on others when the person who is doing the returning arrives on the scene. You can see how these scenes can be embellished for maximum effectiveness. Again, make it realistic, but don't set up impossible situations for our patient group. Tailor these stock scenes to your people and have fun.

After a "stock" scene is run once or twice, with different people taking the part as principals, you can go back to running your social skills group with a livelier bunch.

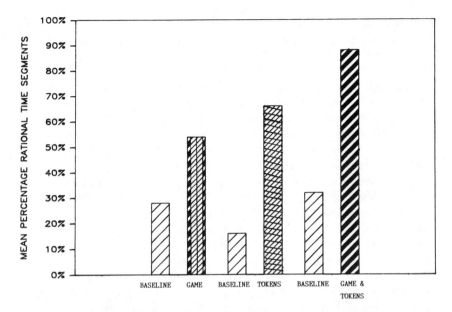

FIGURE 5-1. The mean percentage of one-minute time segments that contained rational and coherent speech in different experimental conditions for three chronic, paranoid schizophrenic patients in a group therapy situation. The game was an adaptation of "The Dating Game" that elicited social awareness and social communication. Very substantial increases in social conversation were produced when token reinforcement was given to the patients contingent upon their conversation as well as when the game was introduced. The greatest amount of spontaneous conversation occurred during the sessions when the game and reinforcement were provided. Tokens were exchanged at the end of the group session for notions, candy, cigarettes, and other tangible rewards.

RESISTANCE AND
REMOTIVATION

Resistance to treatment can be active or passive. The patient can protest loudly and refuse to participate or simply not show up for treatment sessions. A second familiar problem is attendance without attending. The patient is physically present, but doesn't take an active part in what's happening. Motivation to participate is one of the most difficult problems in the rehabilitation of the chronic mental patient. And all too often, the patient drops out entirely and doesn't come back to treatment until the next acute episode of illness.

This shouldn't be so hard to understand. Treatment implies change, and people, no matter what their status, aren't inclined to change their behavior, their level of activity, or their way of thinking about the world. The process of changing behavior and thought has been the subject of more scholarly writings than any other. Change is an unpleasant prospect for the average person, but for the person suffering from a devastating, debilitating mental disorder, it can be frightening.

Remotivating these patients is a constant challenge. How many of us have not been personally affected by patients who have little left in their lives that they enjoy, who are apathetic, apparently depressed, unresponsive, or even oppositional to efforts to kindle a spark of human interest? In social skills training, we have a treatment model that is built on action, reaction, risk taking, and creativity! How can clinicians overcome that sinking sensation, which is like trying to run in deep, wet sand that we often feel while working with the chronic patient? Fortunately, there are a few "tricks of the trade" that really work. These derive not only from clinical folklore but also from careful research findings. Motivational techniques require little in the way of extra material resources, but they do require ingenuity and, above all, that objective trial and error approach that allows you to try a new strategy, to evaluate the results, and to be satisfied with small amounts of progress at a time. Let's look at a few of these remotivation strategies. Your knowledge of your patients and your own creativity will take over where we leave off!

Assuring Attendance

You can't treat the patient if the body isn't there. Spotty attendance is probably the most basic of the "resistance" issues. In fact, the lack of motivation to attend may not be entirely the fault of the patient. Those with whom he or she lives must also be made to see the importance of attendance at treatment sessions and motivated to assist the patient to come to the clinic. Going the extra mile to make contact—by phone or in person—with the patient's relatives, caregivers, or significant others can produce results. Explaining the rationale and importance of the training and putting your heads together on overcoming transportation and other obstacles to attendance can make a big difference.

While we have promoted the advantages of conducting social skills training in groups, you should retain flexibility in using this modality in other formats; for example, for patients with high levels of performance anxiety and social avoidance, having a few initial training sessions in one-to-one therapy might help them gain the comfort and confidence to join a group. In fact, the focus of individual skills training could be on situations that they fear might emerge in the group. Other patients may benefit more from skills training that is offered in a couple or family therapy setting.

Setting the time for the group to meet at a convenient hour may help to overcome resistances to participation that are grounded in real, logistical obstacles. Early evening or late afternoon may be better times for patients who are working. For some tangible aids in getting psychiatric patients to adhere to their social skills training sessions, mental health can take some hints from dental health. Everyone agrees that regular dental checks are necessary, but getting people to overcome the almost universal fear of dental care is as difficult as, well, pulling teeth. Here are some techniques that are used by dentists to improve attendance at appointments. You will find them familiar and useful in getting your patients to show up for their social skills training sessions.

1. *Appointment Cards.* Cards can be official looking or whimsical. They should have the appointment time and place and telephone number clearly displayed. Some dentists have cards that are preprinted and shaped like large theater tickets, with room for the time and date. Whatever the form, we have found that a simple card can be a powerful prompt. Be sure that the patient's family or home operator is aware that appointment cards are given. Encourage the caregivers to remind the patient to tack the card up on a bulletin board or to put it on the refrigerator door with a magnet. The responsibility to remember the session and to take active steps to get there should ultimately be the patient's. At the outset relatives, caregivers, and support people may have to assist in providing some structure and prompting. Later, the prompts should be reduced or faded and the patient rewarded for taking more and more of the responsibility for remembering and going to treatment.

2. *Telephone Calls.* Now commonly used in dentistry and medicine, the telephone call reminding the patient of tomorrow's appointment is cheap insurance against the no-show problem. The time invested in making the calls is paid back in better attendance rates.

3. *Postcards.* Mailing a postcard to the patient is a variation on the appointment card. It has the added benefit of an "official" aura since it arrives in the mail, and it is close to being public communication—the family or home operator is likely to see it before the patient does! Receiving a phone call reminder or postcard reminder to attend a social skills training group is particularly powerful with patients whose social networks have atrophied and hence receive few phone calls or little mail.

4. *Contracts.* Somewhat more formal, but having the advantage of being more precise, is the contractual agreement with the primary goal being increased attendance at treatment. This method is also common in the dental health field, since many dental plans now specify a higher payment by the insured patient for tooth restorations if the patient hasn't been seen for regular checkups.

Behavioral contracts should be worded in positive terms. For example, the contract should specify the rights and privileges that will be gained by the patient for attending training or treatment sessions. The contract should be negotiated with the patient and the family or home operator made fully aware of the contract and its consequences. Clear, step-by-step guidelines for writing behavioral contracts can be found in the manual, *Writing Behavioral Contracts* by W. J. DeRisi and D. Butz (obtainable through Research Press, Box 3177, Dept. H, Champaign, IL 61821).

Rewards for Participation: Coffee, Tea, or Tokens?

For many patients, prompts alone won't sustain attendance and active participation time. Up to now, we have discussed methods of prompting patients and their support people to come to treatment. The rest of the story covers ways to use incentives or rewards for attendance, completion of homework assignments, and active participation.

If you reflect for just a moment on the things that make it more comfortable for you to be in an unfamiliar setting, some possibilities may come to mind. It really doesn't take much to make someone feel wanted and special. Being greeted by name and with genuine warmth is first. How impressed are you when a waiter or maitre d' in a restaurant remembers you and calls you by name? And the room should be set up and ready to go. A lot of last-minute hustle-bustle doesn't contribute to a calm, professional atmosphere. If there are receptionists or clerical staff who guard the door and the waiting room, they should be cautioned and trained to smile and be welcoming to patients as they arrive. Patients may act bizarre, ask repetitive questions, or awkwardly try to strike up conversations, but the brief time they will spend with the office staff should be cordial and warm. An officious, tired secretary can wreak havoc with patients' self-esteem that the clinician works so hard to build.

And then there are refreshments. Even in these days of extreme cost-consciousness, the airlines, banks, high-line department stores, and even no-frills discount stores reward their customers' attendance with a cup of coffee, a free soft drink, a cookie, or even a few salty-sugary peanuts. Provision of light snacks and beverages creates a hospitable atmosphere and may serve to reinforce attendance and participation of patients who find gratification in food.

As a social skills trainer, you can utilize behavioral principles to arrange snacks for good advantage. For example, a little coffee or other beverage can be available as the patients arrive, but the snack food can be brought out at the break or even after the session. A variation on the theme is the use of points or tokens that can be used to purchase the refreshments at the break. Naturally, completion of homework assignments should be rewarded liberally, but partial credit for good attempts should earn points as well.

Points can be given contingent on the level of participation in the actual training itself. Points can be given for assisting in scenes, for offering suggestions, or for carrying out the homework assignments. This approach is a little more complicated, but it takes control of a reinforcer and uses it contingently to shape the behavior of the patients. For those who may still be squeamish about token economies and the use of points and food as reinforcers, there is an interesting sidelight that may make such systems more palatable. In research conducted at the Oxnard (California) Community Mental Health Center, points and token "money" were found to take on great symbolic meaning for patients. That is, the reinforcers that were available in exchange for the tokens appeared to be no more important to the patient than the points themselves. The mere accumulation of these tokens of progress was very satisfying to many patients. Thus, you may want to try a motivational system that simply relies on points or credits for their own sake. It should not be so surprising that any sign of improvement, like the accumulation of points, would be seen as valuable in itself. For our patients—people who are often treated by the world as if they have no value—a tangible sign of their own worth can be precious.

Many of us work in situations where there is little day-to-day feedback of the adequacy of our behavior, but we have learned to get by on very "thin" schedules of social reinforcement. We are treated courteously and with interest by our co-workers, we receive annual performance appraisals or "grades," we get merit increases in our salaries and a gold watch or certificate of recognition after 20 years on the job. So the token system, carried out with respect and good humor, is a very useful tool for nurturing the bruised egos of the psychiatrically disabled.

Token or point systems can use either physical tokens (coin substitutes or specially printed coupons or bills) or checkmarks or punches on a simple card. Some examples are shown in Figure 5-2. Token systems can be made to mimic the world outside the treatment setting, thereby teaching patients the use of real money as an added benefit. There is an extensive literature on the use of these systems, which can be very simple or extremely realistic and complicated. For the purposes of social skills training, a simple system would be best, since you are likely to be busy enough with the actual training steps.

Actual tokens or printed fake money have an advantage for patients needing frequent and immediate reward, since they may be "laid on" for attendance and the many small steps of participation in social skills training. It's easy to drop a token into the patient's hand for such elementary behaviors as keeping eyes open for more than three minutes or for responding to questions, volunteering a rating, or offering to assist in the training. Naturally, each token reward should be accompanied by

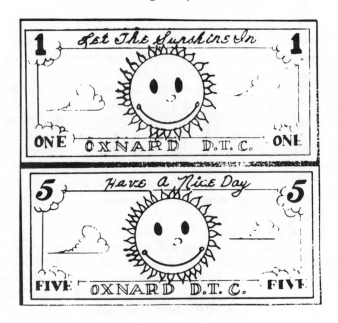

Credit Card

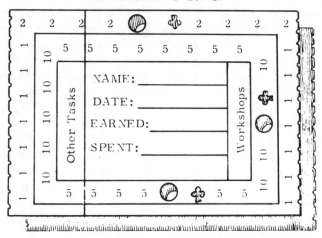

FIGURE 5-2. Examples of coupons or a credit card that can be used as reinforcers for motivating the attendance, participation, and progress of patients in social skills training. Coupons, credits, points, or tokens are given to patients contingent upon the targeted behavior; in turn, these generalized reinforcers are exchanged by patients for a wide variety of tangible rewards.

smiles, appropriate pats, touches, and compliments from the therapist or trainer.

The use of credit cards or punch cards to motivate attendance and participation has a place for motivating patients who can tolerate longer delays in reinforcement. The cards can be marked or punched at the end of the training session with accompanying praise from the therapist for a job well done.

At the Brentwood VA Hospital, chronic mental patients who participate in social skills training receive coupon books that can be redeemed for food and personal objects at the hospital canteen. Volunteer organizations, such as the Military Order of the Purple Heart and the Amvets, contribute money to purchase the canteen books. Patients who attend their social skills training sessions also can obtain reduced-fare bus passes and go on a weekly outing to the beach, amusement park, or movie. The Veterans Administration hospitals also can capitalize upon a motivational system—termed "incentive therapy"—that utilizes real money. By participating in activities—such as social skills training and vocational rehabilitation—that enhance community adaptation and work restoration, patients receive a biweekly paycheck that can be as much as half the minimum hourly wage.

The kinds of rewards for which the earned points or tokens can be exchanged are only limited by your imagination. All the extras that clinical staff have used over the years can be brought into the motivation system. Special trips, a meal at a fast-food place, free tickets coaxed out of the local movie theater manager, and "twofer" tickets to movies or restaurants should all be brought into the action. No-cost activities such as private talks with a favorite staff person or even the opposite—time away from the clinic or hospital—can be used!

The literature on designing and using incentive reward systems in psychiatric settings is rich and varied, and this brief discussion can't take the place of some outside reading on the subject. But the important thing to remember is that you are going to have to take those extra steps to get those customers to come in and buy your social skills products, and keep them coming back for more!

PERSONALIZING THE TRAINING RELATIONSHIP

It is axiomatic that mental health and rehabilitation professionals and paraprofessionals who have good verbal and nonverbal social skills themselves will be effective social skills trainers. In fact, clinicians who are shy, retiring, and cerebral in their approach to patients will be very handicapped in their using the active-directive techniques of social skills training. Preventing and overcoming resistance to social skills training, hence, will depend greatly on the personal qualities of the trainer or therapist.

The enthusiasm that a clinician brings to social skills training can be operationalized by referring to a number of dimensions that are shown in Table 5-1. Facial expression and vocal intonation and delivery are particularly important in communicating enthusiasm. Being out of one's chair and moving close to patients in supportive postures will help to increase one's enthusiasm and will also be contagious to patients. Unfortunately, enthusiasm and charisma are not easily learned by professionals who are characterologically deficient in these attributes. One way to compensate for such deficits is to match as co-therapists a vivacious and enthusiastic clinician with one who is less so.

Even in the absence of charisma, most clinicians have developed or been selected for a personal therapeutic style that includes good listening skills, empathy, genuine human concern, and warmth. However, few clinicians consciously employ specific behaviors that can cumulatively strengthen the therapeutic relationship and thereby minimize resistance. Here are some therapist behaviors that are contributory to the therapeutic alliance and cohesion in social skills training:

1. Before the patient's first visit, give careful directions for finding the way to the place where skills training will take place, for example, by providing a map.
2. Provide equitable physical distance between therapist and patient:
   a. Avoid having desk as a barrier, unless patient prefers interpersonal distance.
   b. Allow a fearful or reluctant patient to sit near the door.
   c. Shake hands with patients *after* the initial visit when it will be more meaningful instead of at the opening introduction.
   d. Greet patients at the door or in the waiting room and walk with them to the door at the end of a session. Say "good-bye" and remind your patients of the next training session.
   e. Use touching and pats on the back with discretion depending upon the patient's comfort and values.
3. Ask permission before using a patient's first name; give each patient the option of how he or she wants to be called and addressed.
4. Apologize if you are late for a session.
5. Show patients where the toilet is located and give them permission to use it whenever needed—even in midst of sessions.
6. Avoid looking at a clock or watch when *patients are talking*.

7. Let occasional sessions go overtime—don't end every session strictly "on the 50-minute hour."
8. Acknowledge your patients' birthdays and anniversaries verbally and possibly with greeting cards.
9. With discretion, greet your patients casually when crossing paths in the community.
10. Use good personal effectiveness nonverbal style—eye contact, resonant voice, fluent and slow speech, spontaneous gestures, leaning toward patients, smiling, and appropriate, reflective facial expressions.
11. Frequently reinforce and acknowledge the mutual interest, concern, and recognition that group members show for one another during the training sessions. This builds cohesion in the training group, thereby facilitating the learning and behavior change process.

PROMOTING PARTICIPATION IN BEHAVIORAL REHEARSAL

One of the key techniques in social skills training is behavioral rehearsal. In behavioral rehearsal, the therapist sets up a clinically relevant interpersonal scene and has the couple or family practice the interaction. Since behavioral rehearsal is such a key element in social skills training therapy, overcoming resistance to practicing emotional expressions and communication patterns is important. It would be very nice, indeed, if all our patients behaved as mature adults and cooperated with our efforts to engage them in behavioral rehearsal. Unfortunately, our patients come to us because they are not mature adults, and their resistance to behavioral rehearsal may be symptomatic of a wide range of affective, cognitive, and social problems. Effective methods of coping with resistance, then, depend upon identifying the sources of the resistance.

With a patient suffering from schizophrenia or severe depression—where biologically mediated symptoms are interfering with attentional, cognitive, and motivational skills required by the behavioral rehearsal—it may be necessary to use medication judiciously for overcoming resistance induced by symptoms. With a spouse of a depressed patient who is paying "lip service" to marital therapy but whose lack of any real interest in improving the marriage is betrayed by half-hearted participation in behavioral rehearsal, a direct exploration may be required of the person's ambivalence. The following suggestions for surmounting resistance to behavioral rehearsal are offered with the assumption that the experienced clinician will use them in the context of a proper evaluation of the types and sources of resistance.

Table 5-1. Enthusiasm in conducting social skills training is a key ingredient in successful outcomes. Especially for patients who have deficits in spontaneity and positive affect, an enthusiastic social skills trainer can produce a contagious effect through social modeling. Motivation for proceeding through arduous and repeated skills training sessions can be transmitted to patients through a spontaneous and enthusiastic trainer. The following behavioral descriptions of different levels of verbal and nonverbal enthusiasm can help to improve your own impact as a social skills trainer. The following material first appeared in the June 1981 issue of *Practical Applications of Research*, a newsletter published quarterly by Phi Delta Kappa, the professional education fraternity. It is adapted here by permission.

| | Enthusiasm Level | | |
	Low	Medium	High
Vocal Delivery	Monotone, minimum inflections, little variation in speech, poor articulation.	Pleasant variations of pitch, volume, and speed; good articulation.	Frequent, varied, and sudden changes of pitch
Eyes	Looks dull or bored; seldom opens eyes wide or raises eyebrows; avoids eye contact; often maintains a blank stare.	Appears interested; occasionally lighting up, shining, opening wide.	Appears as dancing, snapping, shining, lighting up frequently, opening wide, eyebrows raised; maintains eye contact while avoiding staring.
Gestures	Seldom moves arms out toward person or object; never uses sweeping movements; keeps arms at side or folded, rigid.	Often points, occasional sweeping motion using body, head, arms, hands and face; maintains steady pace of gesturing.	Quick and demonstrative movements of body, head, arms, hands, and face.

188

Body Movement	Seldom moves from one spot, or from sitting to standing position; sometimes paces nervously.	Moves freely, slowly, and steadily.	Large body movements, swings around, walks rapidly, changes pace; unpredictable and energetic; natural body movements.
Facial Expression	Appears deadpan, expressionless, or frowns; little smiling; lips closed.	Agreeable; smiles frequently; looks pleased, happy, or sad if situation called for.	Appears vibrant, demonstrative; shows many expressions; broad smile; quick, sudden changes in expression.
Word Selection	Mostly nouns, few descriptions or adjectives; simple or trite.	Some descriptors, adjectives, or repetition of the same ones.	Highly descriptive, many adjectives, great variety.
Acceptance of Ideas and Feelings	Little indication of acceptance or encouragement; may ignore patient's feelings or ideas.	Accepts ideas and feelings; praises or clarifies; some variations in response, but frequently repeats same ones.	Quick to accept, praise, encourage, or clarify; many variations in response; vigorous nodding of head when agreeing.
Overall Energy Level	Lethargic; appears inactive, dull, or sluggish.	Appears energetic and demonstrative sometimes, but mostly maintains an even level.	Exuberant; high degree of energy and vitality; highly demonstrative.

Acknowledging Sources of Resistance

Many times, resistance can be quickly dissolved by the therapist simply reflecting back the emotions, inhibitions, and anxieties that are behind the negativism. This is particularly effective when mild anxiety or embarrassment are at the root of the resistance. Straightforward performance anxiety can often get in the way of direct practice of interpersonal scenes—acknowledgment dilutes the anxiety, gives "permission" for experiencing discomfort, and prompts confidence and rapport with the therapist. It is important not to overreact to resistance by offering elaborate psychological interpretations that may only serve to reinforce them. Simple and direct acknowledgment should be quickly followed by prompts to participate in small steps.

Carol, deciding she wanted to practice assertive skills with her parents who were overly protective and excessively concerned with her whereabouts, blocked when she was asked to try a scene from her home life in a "dry run" rehearsal. She was noticeably tense and anxious, which the trainer realized was disrupting her performing the scene.

Therapist: Carol, I can understand your being uptight going through this difficult scene, but let's give it a try even though you may be uncomfortable. After you practice it and watch others demonstrating it, you'll feel more confident.

Carol: You mean it's OK to be nervous?

Therapist: Sure, it's natural. In fact, being nervous tells us that this is an important situation for you to be able to handle. So let's give it a try and tolerate being anxious for now.

Modeling for the Resistant Patient

Borrowing from psychodramatic techniques, the clinician can "double" for the patient who is reluctant to rehearse a scene. By doubling or providing an auxiliary ego, some of the pressure for initiating or processing an interpersonal problem can be taken off the resistant patient who can repeat, word for word, the phrases spoken by the "double."

Another use of modeling is to have the patient observe the therapist taking the patient's role and then asking the patient to criticize, revise, or elaborate on the therapist's performance. This gives the patient a chance to learn vicariously through observing the therapist and to become task involved. With very anxious and inhibited patients, it may be necessary to allow the patient to watch others engage in behavioral rehearsal for a session or two before prompting active participation on the patient's part.

Shaping Participation in Small Steps

A sensitive therapist can subtly slip the resistant patient into rehearsing by asking the patient to describe in concrete, graphic details what generally happens in the actual problem situations. The patient will usually volunteer descriptions of who did what to whom after which the therapist can prompt. "When he said that to you, you said _____(pause)_____?" Even getting a patient to take the first-person position during a single interaction is a step toward full participation in rehearsing a scene.

Other ways of breaking down the rehearsal into smaller responses include setting up a brief and emotionally nonthreatening scene that has no "heavy" personal loading for the patient. Therefore, in trying to gain the participation of a resistant adolescent, it would be counterproductive to invite a rehearsal of a scene dealing with parental confrontation over marijuana use; instead, it would be wise to start with a mundane scene, such as how family members greet each other or say goodbye to each other. Another use of shaping through approximations is to ask the resistant patient member to take the role of a different person inside or outside of the family circle and play that person's part in a behavioral rehearsal. Once some practice in another person's role has been carried out, anxiety has usually diminished to the point where the patient can then rehearse his or her own role.

Using Group Process

One of the many advantages in conducting social skills training in groups is the opportunity to overcome resistance to behavioral rehearsal. In a group, the therapist has the option of beginning the rehearsals with the most enthusiastic and cooperative patients or with those who are "veterans" of behavioral rehearsal. This capitalizes on their modeling impact on resistant and shy group members. Group process also promotes cohesion, which has a relaxing effect on inhibited group members. In a group, the therapist can allow new or resistant members simply to observe the more active members. As they watch the others getting involved and gaining the therapist's interest and feedback, the most reluctant patients will be motivated to participate. Asking the more resistant patient to give verbal suggestions and feedback to other participating members also serves as an approximation to their subsequent, more active involvement in the treatment process.

Strategic Ploys

In undercutting resistance that might otherwise develop, an astute therapist will also spend time on catharsis and determining the patient's reasons for coming for help. Sufficient opportunity for ventilating feelings and concerns—even at the risk of temporarily reinforcing maladaptive tendencies—is important to provide *before* engaging the patient in goal-setting and structured therapy. If the patient feels he or she has not been "heard" before therapy commences, counterproductive complaining and foot dragging will often occur during the therapy.

Demonstrating your competence to the new patient or group of patients being readied for social skills training will undercut later resistance. Competence is conveyed by a cogent and comprehensible rationale for the training and how it will benefit the patients with their problems. Competence is also demonstrated by personalizing the goals and methods of training to the specific needs and concerns of each patient. For example, a patient who has not dated with the opposite sex for five years needs to be steered toward nonthreatening heterosocial situations, such as conversing with sales clerks or persons in service agencies. Through experiencing initial success with these low-demand interactions in the training sessions and homework assignments, the patient quickly gains confidence in the therapist or trainer and is likely to participate actively and positively in future sessions.

The use of paradoxical and other subtle methods can be useful in gaining the compliance of patients to therapeutic instructions for behavioral rehearsal and homework assignments. It should be emphasized, however, that therapists require some finesse and experience to use these interventions effectively. Some of the strategic interventions, useful in eliciting the cooperation of a patient, are

1. Establish a "response set" for compliance and cooperation through initially making small requests that can be easily agreed to. Thus, after agreeing to pass an ashtray, use a different chair, and write a list of complaints, the patient has already begun to cooperate and may be more likely to respond favorably to larger requests in the future.
2. "Join" with the patient's resistance—identify with patient's concerns and thereby avoid a power struggle. For example, tell a fearful patient, "It's common to feel anxious and tense when starting social skills training. In time, you'll be ready to participate."
3. Emphasize positive behavior and downplay resistance in talking with patient; for example, say, "Despite your reluctance to being involved in social skills training, you *are* here today and have made an effort to get help."

4. Establish *this therapy* as distinct and different from the other therapies which have failed in the past.
5. Give permission to engage in noncooperation and noncompliance.
   a. Instruct patient actually to *practice* being resistant or silent. Say "It's all right to just sit in your chair. You'll learn a lot by just watching others practice."
   b. Schedule their symptomatic behavior; for example, instruct a patient who tends to resist active participation to take a "rest" from training every other session and simply observe the others in the group practice.
   c. Introduce an "ordeal" as an accompaniment to resistant behavior; for example, patients who have temper tantrums or symptomatic episodes can be asked to walk around the block until "feeling more calm" and then return to the skills training session.
6. Predict resistance; thus, patients starting a group can be told, "At some time or another you'll have trouble rehearsing in the sessions and will want to avoid completing homework assignments."
7. Provide a choice or option for the patient to decide on, either of which is therapeutic; for example, "You can either practice accepting compliments from your roommate or criticism from your work supervisor. Which scene do you choose?"
8. Emphasize a worse alternative to behavioral rehearsal; for example, "Instead of rehearsing a situation today, you can take responsibility for writing out everybody's homework assignment cards."

TRAINING DISTRACTIBLE AND THOUGHT-DISORDERED PATIENTS

To benefit from the social skills training methods described in Chapters 3 and 4, patients must be able to pay attention to features of the training situation for 30–90 minutes. In addition, patients need the capacity for understanding instructions without a great deal of repetition and for making themselves understood to others. These basic cognitive and verbal skills are not available to a minority of patients with chronic schizophrenia—perhaps 10–15 percent of all schizophrenic patients— who suffer from severe forms of distractibility and incoherence. These patients require a much more intensive, focused, and individualized form of training for basic verbal and attentional skills, akin to the language development techniques that have proved effective in teaching mute and echolalia autistic and retarded persons to speak.

A social skills training method for thought-disordered psychiatric patients has been developed and evaluated that aims at focusing the patient's attention on the relevant steps and cues in the training procedure while minimizing demands on cognitive abilities. The attention-focusing procedure is characterized by multiple, discrete, relatively short training trials. A closely structured training situation minimizes distractibility by carefully manipulating the teaching components in each trial. This procedure has been used to train highly distractible institutionalized chronic schizophrenic patients in conversational skills.

While roleplaying, corrective feedback, modeling, prompting, and reinforcement are important elements, the attention-focusing model is distinguished by the controlled and sequential presentation of the training components. The trainer initiates a conversation with the patient by making a statement. If the patient makes a correct response, he or she is praised, and the response is sometimes reinforced with something to eat or drink. If a correct response is not forthcoming, the trainer implements a prompt sequence. The patient is praised if he or she responds appropriately. The trainer presents the same statement to the patient until he or she responds correctly several times in succession. Then the patient is trained in responses to new conversational statements.

The following is an example of attention focusing with a chronic schizophrenic patient named Sue who has been hospitalized continuously for 15 years. She has been described as socially isolated and highly distractible. In an individual session, a therapist and an aide named Tom are training Sue in how to compliment others.

Tom: I just bought this shirt yesterday.
Sue: (no response)
Therapist: Sue, give Tom a compliment.
Sue: (no response)
Therapist: One compliment you can give is "That's a nice shirt."
Sue: (no response)
Tom: I just bought this shirt yesterday.
Sue: (no response)
Therapist: One compliment you can give is "That's a nice shirt."
Sue: That's a nice shirt.
Tom: Thank you very much.
Therapist: Very good, Sue, that is a nice compliment.
Tom: I just bought this shirt yesterday.
Sue: (no response)
Therapist: Sue, give Tom a compliment.
Sue: I like your shirt.

Tom: I'm glad you like it.
Therapist: That is a very good compliment, Sue.
Tom: I just bought this shirt yesterday.
Sue: That is a nice shirt.
Tom: Oh, thank you, Sue.
Therapist: Excellent, Sue. That's a nice compliment. Have a little soda.
Tom: I just bought this shirt yesterday.
Sue: That is a nice shirt.
Tom: Thank you, Sue.
Therapist: Very, very good. Sue. Now you are making nice compliments.

Typically patients are taught to make 8 to 12 alternative responses, or exemplars, in each domain of conversational skills. Steps are then taken to promote transfer of training to other appropriate situations if generalization does not occur spontaneously. This model has been validated by training a group of patients in three conversational skills—asking questions, giving compliments, and making requests to engage in activities with others. Results indicated that this highly structured procedure was effective for training social skills in withdrawn, incoherent, low-functioning, chronic psychiatric patients.

SUMMARY

You should assume that patients are doing the best they can in social skills training and therefore resistance to change exists for good reasons. The therapist can build motivation to participate in social skills training even for very difficult patients.

The best cure for resistance is to prevent it. How a person is invited to join is critical: You should provide a rationale, have the primary therapist or referring clinician be primed to give prospective patients some favorable orientation in advance of the referral, and give the patient an explanatory orientation as with using the kind of brochure describing the process found in Appendix A to this guidebook. The whole idea is to build favorable, but realistic, expectations.

Good planning will prevent resistance. By this we mean that participation will be assured if you have gone through a thorough needs assessment; arrived at some relevant goals and objectives and built expectations of attaining them; blocked efforts to defeat treatment or the therapist; and planned how the training should proceed for that patient. Careful orientation and attainable objectives are easy to design because of the down-to-earth and direct methods that are used.

Even difficult patients respond to these steps, especially if the therapist is flexible and is willing to settle for minimal participation at first. Avoiding power struggles requires foresight and a knowledge of how to proceed before the situation deteriorates. Concentrating on the problem-solving process can prevent or minimize disruption in training and in the real patient's world assignments. Having patients who are reluctant to participate first observe others rehearsing and then making small but slowly increasing requests for practicing is very effective in overcoming social anxiety, inhibitions, and negativism. Cajoling, arguing, and rational efforts at persuasion are much less effective methods.

Patients whose skills are very deficient or regressed require a slightly different approach, but the therapist still has to settle for small but increasing bits of participation by laying on small but increasing demands. The deficient patient must be taught the paralinguistic and nonverbal elements of social skills before going on to learn problem solving, accurate social perception, and social judgment.

Use a variety of "stock" or "canned" exercises to maintain interest and energy in social skills training. These exercises use exaggerated action, high levels of activity, and humor, and permit patients to step out of their personal roles and concerns. Warm-up exercises are important to set the pace of the session. Increasing the level of activity at the beginning of a session can prevent losing the group's attentiveness later on. More than just entertainment, these exercises allow a real-time assessment of how patients are feeling and behaving right now. Very current information about skill training needs can be gotten using these apparently innocuous, but enjoyable exercises.

Motivation is one of the most critical problems in the treatment of the chronic patient. Treatment encourages change and change is difficult for everyone. It is especially frightening for the mentally ill. Appointment cards, telephone calls, mailed postcards, and behavioral contracts should be used as prompts to increase attendance. A rewarding environment can be constructed by employing a point or token system, with liberal use of social approval and interaction along with simple refreshments. By linking the rewards to effort, participation, and accomplishment, the investment in these incentives will pay off in a better attendance and a higher degree of participation. Volunteer and other community service organizations can be tapped to defray the costs of refreshments or other incentives. No-cost items should be used: Time with a special staff person or even time off from a session are examples of effective rewards. Personalizing the training is also a potent source of motivation.

The therapist behaviors or competencies described in this chapter can cement the therapeutic alliance and group cohesion in social skills training. Getting patients to engage in behavioral rehearsal can be a challenge. Acknowledging the sources of resistance, modeling and "doubling," shaping participation in small steps, asking resistant patients to give feedback to others, and other strategic ploys are often necessary to help patients to rehearse. Attention-focusing may be used to increase the meaningful participation of seriously thought-disordered or otherwise distractible patients.

Appendix A

Social Skills Training for Psychiatric Patients "Orientation for Patients"

This "Orientation" to social skills training has been prepared for patients and clients newly referred to or just beginning this type of therapy. It is advisable to duplicate this "Orientation" and use it as a handout to new patients to help acclimate them to the structured and educational methods they will encounter. "Orientation" will promote favorable and realistic expectations for the subsequent experience in training and will reduce performance anxiety and discomfort during the first few sessions.

ORIENTATION TO
SOCIAL SKILLS TRAINING
FOR PATIENTS AND CLIENTS

Welcome to Social Skills Training! We want to give you an idea of what it's all about to help you get into this kind of treatment activity. We want you to know just what will happen, what to expect, and how you will benefit from Social Skills Training. First, let's describe what we want to accomplish: Social Skills Training helps people improve the way they communicate their feelings, needs, and wishes to others. It also helps them respond to other people's feelings, needs, and wishes more effectively. The result is that you can get what you want more often and, just as important, you can avoid doing things that others want you to do—but you don't!

One good way ι describe how all this works is to show you some of the questions that people ask most often about Social Skills Training. You may have some more questions of your own, and you can ask them of your therapist, doctor, or social skills trainer.

What Exactly Is Taught
in Social Skills Training?

We work on some of the simple things that make for good communication: How to choose the right words and expressions for specific occasions; how to accurately sense the other person's feelings and needs; how loud or soft your voice is; how well you look at people when you are talking to them; how well your facial expression matches your mood, whether happy or sad, interested or bored; and your posture and hand gestures when you are talking to other people. In Social Skills Training, learning to use the most effective words and phrases is important, but even more important is learning *how* to put our messages across effectively.

Do Specific Communication Skills
Really Make a Difference?

Absolutely! As a matter of fact, the WAY people communicate is just as important as what it is that they say. Social Skills Training isn't like most forms of group therapy, because we don't sit around and talk about problems. We actually *try out ways of solving problems* with other people. We practice them and then we try them out in real-life situations.

Will I Have to Get up in Front of
Strangers in a Group and Perform?

You'll be with about four to ten other people—a small group. But no, you won't be expected to practice new skills until you're ready and willing. You'll be politely introduced to the other members of the group by the trainer or therapist and will hear, first hand, about the steps used in Social Skills Training. At first, you'll be asked to watch, then to help other people by giving your opinion on how they do in the session. Then you can help in the actual training for others by taking the part of people in their lives with whom they want to communicate. Only when you're comfortable with the procedures, how the training works, and with the people in the group will you be asked to work on some of your own skills.

What Actually Does Each Person
DO in This Training?

As I've said, we DON'T do a lot of talking and discussing. We DO a lot of demonstrating, actually showing how you can improve communication with others. It's fine to describe the problems we're having, and even to understand why we keep having problems, but changing for the better usually requires more active learning by observing others, getting instructions and coaching, and practicing new skills. In Social Skills Training, you can learn a lot by watching how other people would handle problem situations, and then you can try out what you've observed. Coaching, like that given by a movie director or sports coach, will be given by the trainer or therapist to help you improve. You'll get a lot of good hints on what you can do better, but you won't get any unpleasant criticism. No one makes fun of anything in Social Skills Training—it's not allowed. In fact, you'll get loads of praise and encouragement for even small steps you take. You'll be surprised how quickly you improve this way.

What Good Will Social Skills Training Do for Me?

Social Skills Training will give you a lot more confidence in dealing with many different kinds of people—people who can make you feel uncomfortable or angry or sad or even bored. You will be able to identify what they are doing to make you feel that way, and then you can use some new skills to change that. We all have difficulty dealing with certain people. Sometimes it's a parent or spouse or friend; sometimes it's bosses, co-workers, or people who work in stores or restaurants. And sometimes it's policemen or teachers. And of course, sometimes it's people of the opposite sex. We can all use some ideas on how we can deal with others better!

If You Don't Criticize, How Do You Tell People What They Are Doing Wrong?

Well, the first thing we do is tell people what they did RIGHT. Then we give suggestions on how to improve. That's a rule in the sessions. And we never break that rule. You've heard the term "constructive criticism." That means to teach people how to improve their interactions and exchanges with others. Instructions, coaching, and demonstrations by other group members and by the trainer all combine to give you momentum to improve your communication skills.

How Do You Apply What's Practiced in the Training Sessions?

By doing homework. Everyone gets a real-life assignment to carry out before the next session. But it's not like school homework. You don't write papers or do things like that. Instead, your real-life assignment may be to go to a company and bring back one of their job application forms, or to ask a friend to go shopping for clothing with you. Whatever it is, it's related to the situation you practiced in the last training session and to the personal goals you've set for yourself. Later on, the assignments get harder, but they'll always be something you've practiced and feel confident you can do.

How Will I Remember to Do the Homework?

You'll always get a little card with the assignment written on it. That helps you remember what you are supposed to do. Sometimes you'll be asked to have someone sign the card to show that you actually had a conversation or went someplace. Actually, the homework assignments are a lot of fun.

Sometimes you'll be asked to bring back a souvenir from your assignment, like the blank job application, or a theater ticket, or a cash register receipt. One person had an assignment to go to the beach with some friends and bring back a little sand in a sandwich bag!

Don't You Have to Get Your Confidence up to Do This Kind of Thing?

Not really. Most people think they have to FEEL good first before they can learn to DO something new. As a matter of fact, Social Skills Training is designed to BUILD CONFIDENCE. We've found that you become more confident by doing this kind of practice, rather than trying to "psych yourself up" first. It's just like riding a bicycle, driving a car, or using a computer. You can read about it and think about it and talk to other people about it, but the only way you can learn to do it well is by doing it. And when people start practicing, they begin to feel better and they gain confidence in themselves.

If you have any other questions about Social Skills Training, just ask your trainer, therapist, or doctor. We are sure that you will enjoy your participation and improve your life.

Appendix B

Social Skills Training for Psychiatric Patients "Introduction for Professionals"

The purpose of this introduction is to give you a clear picture of Social Skills Training so that you will be able to convey to patients whom you wish to refer to this type of treatment, what they can expect, and how they will benefit from this type of therapy. We recommend that you read through this introduction before referring a patient to Social Skills Training. Getting a realistic picture of Social Skills Training will help you make effective referrals and will ensure that your patient will "connect" and "engage" successfully in the training. It would be desirable for you to read or summarize this introduction to your patient and be prepared to answer your patient's questions before the referral is made.

This "Introduction for Professionals" can be duplicated by those conducting Social Skills Training and sent to mental health and rehabilitation professionals who might have patients who could benefit from this type of treatment. Circulating this introduction will both increase the number of your referrals and improve the quality and appropriateness of the referrals. You may wish to modify the introduction to enhance its fit with the type and thrust of the Social Skills Training program you are providing.

INTRODUCTION TO SOCIAL SKILLS TRAINING FOR PROFESSIONALS REFERRING PATIENTS AND CLIENTS

Social Skills Training helps people to improve the way they communicate their feelings, emotions, needs, and desires to others. It also provides training for better ways of responding to other people by knowing how to tune in and be more sensitive and accurate in understanding what others are trying to say. Since stress and problems often build up in the relationships patients have with friends, acquaintances, relatives, and co-workers, Social Skills Training can teach them how to go about solving problems in their everyday life. This will reduce stress as well as increase their daily satisfaction and contentment.

What Are Social Skills?

Social skills are the ways we get across to others how we feel, what we want, the information we need, facts and opinions, and the changes we want in others. Social skills are necessary for getting our material needs met—such as finding a job, getting along with co-workers and supervisors, locating a place to live, getting help from social agencies and health care facilities, and using our money carefully in stores. In almost every walk of life, we must achieve our needs for money, for food, for shelter, and other living needs by communicating effectively with other people. Social skills are also required for meeting our social and emotional needs with friends and relatives. All of us need a sympathetic ear at certain times when we're down on our luck and we also need affection and fun. These "warm fuzzies" in life are obtained by being personally effective in our relationships with friends and family. So, you can see that social skills are the tools we use to meet our full human potential.

In Social Skills Training, we concentrate on elements of communication that are often overlooked. The words we use are important, but even more important than the specific word can be *how* we put our message across. What's involved in *how* we use our words? Simple things, and so obvious that you might miss them. The way you hold your body, how you use your eyes, your hand gestures, your tone of voice, the volume of your voice, and your facial expressions are elements that make or break a message. Smiling when you're angry, mumbling when you want to be "perfectly clear," looking away when you should be steadfast in your irresistible gaze—all these are extremely important. But they don't come naturally; they are learned. If they can be learned, then they can be taught—efficiently, directly, in Social Skills Training.

Since most of our human needs, whether for material things like a job or a home or for emotional support and affection, must be satisfied through contacts and interactions with other people, almost any problem that you might have could be dealt with in Social Skills Training. Here are some examples from actual patients and clients who have profited from Social Skills Training.

- A student who was unable to make friends
- A husband who couldn't express affection to his wife
- A woman who was afraid to ask her landlord to make repairs to her apartment
- A laborer who was unable to stand up to his boss' unfair criticism
- An alcoholic who had trouble refusing invitations from friends to drink
- A young man living at home who needed more privacy but wasn't able to explain his needs to his parents
- A foreman in a factory who had great difficulty confronting his workers with their poor performance and who was developing anxiety and depression
- A mother of four children who was depressed and overburdened by childrearing responsibilities, but who was not able to ask her husband for help in disciplining and managing their children
- A person who had serious side effects from his medication but who didn't know how to get his concerns across to his doctor

Common goals that people have achieved in Social Skills Training include making friends, starting conversations, asking for help from a professional person, succeeding at a job interview, solving family problems, improving a marriage or friendship, coping with criticism and anger, and getting discharged from the hospital.

What to Expect in Social Skills Training

Before beginning Social Skills Training, you should have some idea of what to expect. The first time you attend, you may not be asked to do anything more than observe and introduce yourself. You may watch other people rehearsing their skills and planning ways to meet their personal goals. This will give you some ideas for setting your own goals and will demonstrate how the training works. If you choose, you may take part during that first session, but it is not required. You may be given the chance to help another person practice a skill by taking the role of someone whom that person is trying to communicate with. Since you will be new to Social Skills Training, the therapist or another "veteran" member of the group will explain the purposes of Social Skills Training and how the session is run. Getting into a new situation, like attending Social Skills Training, is always accompanied by a little apprehension or nervousness, especially when you are dealing with some of your personal problems. Expect to be a little tense the first few times you come to Social Skills Training—it's normal and a little like swimming. Once you're in the water, it's comfortable; getting there is half the agony.

Some people are a little nervous about practicing situations from their lives in Social Skills Training, but this subsides very quickly. One reason is that the individual practice sessions or "scenes" are very short, and seldom last more than two minutes. Things happen so fast and you are so busy that there is practically no time to get nervous. And soon, as you begin to pick up new skills, this will become the most enjoyable part of your training. Also, a little nervousness can even be a good thing. Even the best clergy, actors, salespersons, and lawyers admit to feeling a bit nervous before a big event. The observer doesn't see it, however. He or she sees the confident, capable, effective person convincing others to see things the way he or she sees them.

Last, but of equal importance to feedback and rehearsal, are real-life assignments. As each new skill is learned, you will receive assignments to be completed at home, in stores, in restaurants, or on the job.

How Does Social Skills Training Work?

More like going to a class than taking therapy, Social Skills Training uses educational methods. While the training can take place in one-to-one individual counseling or therapy and also in marital and family therapy, it is most often done in small groups. We have found that small groups are the best way to learn social skills because people pick up skills quicker, learn from each other, get more practice, and really enjoy the whole process. Social Skills Trainers can be doctors, nurses, psychologists, social workers, counselors, and other professionals who have had the necessary training and experience. You will notice that your Social Skills Trainer will be very active and direct, giving instructions and feedback to help the learning process move along.

One basic training element is called rehearsal or roleplaying. Practicing the situations that pose problems for you in a "pretend it's real" fashion, enable you to learn new and improved ways to deal with these situations. You and the trainer will design the rehearsals or roleplays so they meet your needs for learning social skills. Remember, "the soul of learning is repetition," so repeatedly practicing your skills, trying them out on a variety of different people, watching others show how they would handle the same situation, and then using the skills in real life are the ways to build your confidence and abilities.

After you and the therapist or trainer have selected a goal—which is always some type of person-to-person situation where you want to succeed in meeting your needs—the action begins. For example, a young woman may be rehearsing her skills at telling her boss, in a nice but firm way, that she would like him to speak to her in a normal tone rather than yelling. She will pick a person from the group who resembles her boss to play her boss in the rehearsal or roleplay. She will tell that person how her boss acts and what she wants to accomplish. The two will then rehearse the scene very briefly, perhaps for only a minute, but certainly for less than three minutes. Immediate positive feedback will be given to the young woman for her initial efforts and constructive suggestions will be made for improving her communication to the boss. Another person, either a patient or the therapist or co-trainer, may be called upon to demonstrate an improved alternative way to play the scene with the boss. The young woman will watch the "model" and then rehearse the scene again, this time trying to incorporate into her own style some of the improvements demonstrated by the "model." During the rerun or second rehearsal, the trainer will be close to her, signaling and whispering encouragement and suggestions to help her learn to improve her communication.

Does Social Skills Training Really Work?

Research carried out over the past two decades has clearly documented the effectiveness of Social Skills Training in teaching people to improve their ability to communicate, obtain their needs in daily life, and express their emotions. Social Skills Training works for people with a variety of emotional or mental problems, physical or medical problems, and for those without disorders or illnesses. By equipping persons with the ability to get across their points of view and desires, Social Skills Training strengthens the personality and protects against stress and illness.

You may doubt that you can learn to express yourself effectively because you lack self-confidence. That may be true to a certain degree, but the point to understand is that YOU FEEL THE WAY YOU ACT, not the reverse. Act assertively (We'll show you how) and you'll feel more confident; act afraid and timid and you'll be afraid. In Social Skills Training, we feel that the participating patient or client is always doing the very best he or she can do. We don't expect you to come to the training session full of energy and motivation; in fact, the training procedures help to build energy, confidence and motivation in you—through taking small steps toward your longer-term goals. If you encounter difficulties applying the skills you learn in the session to your real life, we will be there to assist and to figure out ways of helping you succeed. All we need is your willingness to learn and to experiment with some new ways of expressing yourself.

Everyone can benefit from coaching and practice in some area of social functioning. Salespersons, executives, clergy, and entertainers all take training to improve the way they communicate with others. There is nothing insincere or phony about learning to be more effective, more persuasive or less passive, less put-upon. When a student picks up a paintbrush in an art class, the skills he or she brings to that first lesson are just the raw materials to be improved, sharpened, and refined. No one would argue that the student's abilities are "part of his personality" and somehow fixed and unchangeable. The student may never become another Renoir or Picasso, but it is certain that most people's art skills can be vastly improved with instruction.

So, too, can the way we deal with other people be greatly improved with training. We can learn—all of us—to be more effective with the people we deal with every day. Each of us has some special skills that could use some improvement, but without feedback and instructions from others, we don't change, we just go on, year after year, making the same mistakes. A great poet had part of the answer when he said that it would be a great gift if we could "see ourselves as others see us." Feedback is an important part of Social Skills Training because we get very careful, very specific information on our performance from the instructions and from other trainees. The feedback is always positive, always constructive, and never embarrassing.

Don't we get "feedback" every day—from our relatives, friends, and fellow workers? That's true, but it is too often a jumble of criticism, anger, and sweet talk. None of it will give us the information we need in a way that we can accept and use. When we are criticized or face someone who is hostile, we get defensive and either retreat or attack. In any event, we feel badly later. Well-meaning, friendly people either can't, or feel too embarrassed, to help us and are afraid of hurting our feelings. They assure us that we're just fine, that we're doing everything as well as can be expected. Some relatives nag, carping and snapping until we turn them off or snap back. Supervisors gripe, employees grumble, friends smile, relatives argue, and we desperately try to pick out the true signals about ourselves. No wonder it's difficult! In Social Skills Training you get straight, constructive, easy-to-take information about the way others see you, presented in a way that you can use to improve your social and communication skills.

Completing Real-Life Assignments

Practicing social and communication skills is important for learning to occur, but putting the newly learned skills to use in your real-life situations is the "bottom line" or best way to make the skills a part of you. After you demonstrate some proficiency in the rehearsal or roleplay, you will be given an assignment to actually perform the skills you've practiced with the person or persons in the real situations. Assignments usually are very similar to what was practiced in the skills training session, so you will have already gained some confidence before putting them to use. Some examples of homework assignments, related to the examples of problems described at the beginning of this brochure, are:

- Start three brief, one-minute conversations with other students in your class, asking them how they like the teacher.
- When you come home from work, tell your wife how glad you are to see her.
- Tell your landlord that you realize he or she is busy, but you really need and would appreciate his or her help in repairing the faucet in your kitchen.
- Let your boss know you want to hear when you are not meeting his or her expectations, but that it would be more helpful if he or she could tell you specifically how to improve.
- Tell your parents that you enjoy spending time with them, but your privacy is important and you need time alone to relax and keep your stress level down.

In Social Skills Training, you will receive an assignment card that reminds you what you need to accomplish between sessions. On the other side of the card are some cues for being personally effective. Use the cards, refer to them, and bring them back to the next session because you will be asked by your therapist to report on how your assignment went. Trying out new skills will feel awkward at first, but remember that trying anything new the first few times feels awkward until you gain confidence. Remember how awkward you felt the first few times you rode a two-wheeled bicycle, used roller skates, or drove a car? As you continue to put your newly learned communication skills into real-life practice, you will gradually feel better and more comfortable.

Rehearsal, feedback, models, practice, and assignments: All these elements work together to make you a more effective communicator and to improve the quality of your personal relations. Welcome to Social Skills Training!

Appendix C
Checklist for Competence in Conducting Social Skills Training

The competency criteria listed below are the behavioral skills that need to be used by therapists, trainers, and counselors who wish to effectively conduct Social Skills Training, either with groups, families, or individuals. The list of criteria can be used as a self-assessment guide by both neophyte and experienced clinicians who are interested in employing Social Skills Training techniques. The highly structured techniques and educational skills require the trainer to adopt the role of "coach" or "teacher" rather than "traditional therapist." Clinicians are urged to master the structured and active techniques so that their own personal styles and qualities can be integrated in a procedure that will enhance the impact of Social Skills Training.

- Promote favorable expectations through clear orientation of patients.
- Move the patient from a general problem to a specific scene with limited goals.
- Simulate the real-life situation by choosing appropriate props for the setting and roleplayers for the scene.
- Engage patient in behavioral rehearsal.
- Identify behavioral assets and deficits and suggest constructive alternatives from the "dry run" or initial behavioral rehearsal.
- Elicit and teach "receiving" skills (i.e., accurate social perception) and "processing" skills (i.e., generating alternatives for problem solving).
- Focus on nonverbal and paralinguistic elements of emotional expressiveness as well as on verbal content and timing.
- Use modeling to teach more effective, alternative emotional expressiveness and social skills.

- Be active and directive in coaching and prompting desired changes, especially during the "re-run" of the behavioral rehearsal.
- Give positive feedback for even small improvements and effort—use a "shaping attitude" whereby incremental approximations to needed social skills are abundantly reinforced.
- Solicit positive feedback for participating patient from co-therapists and other members in the group.
- Get physically close to the practicing patient for support and coaching.
- Ignore or suppress inappropriate or deviant behavior if and when it occurs—maintain a favorable learning atmosphere.
- Keep the scenes and roleplaying brief and crisp—use "dry run," modeling, "re-run" format.
- Give specific, attainable, and functional assignments.
- Give feedback and approval for effort and success in completing assignments.
- Employ problem-solving in helping patients to reach their short- and long-term goals.

Appendix D
Rathus Assertiveness Schedule

This self-report inventory has been studied to attest to its reliability and validity. It is effective in distinguishing groups of clinical and sub-clinical populations and is sensitive to the effects of social skills training. This schedule can be used to identify goals for social skills training as well as to measure progress over time. Users of this schedule should be aware of the possible mismatch between a patient's observed social behavior and the self-reported responses on the schedule by the patient. Discrepancies may be useful information about differences between a patient's performance in real-life situations and his or her perception of that performance.

Be cautioned that some patients will have difficulty with the readability of this inventory. You may have to revise the wording to make it more comprehensible or administer the inventory as an interview to ensure that the patient understands the questions. Normative data indicate that persons without psychiatric disorders have average total scores around the mid-point "O" level while patients with schizophrenia score significantly lower. Patients with anxiety and depressive disorder score in the range between psychotics and normals.

The total score is obtained by adding numerical responses to each item after changing the sign of the asterisked items that need to be reversed. The reversal procedure is done to reduce the tendency for social desirability to bias the results. A shorter version of the schedule can be administered by using only the items that are italicized. More information can be obtained regarding this schedule in the following publications.

Rathus, S. A. (1973). A 30-item schedule for assessing assertive behavior. *Behavior Therapy,* 4, 398–406.

Rathus, S. A., & Nevid, J. S. (1977). Concurrent validity of the 30-item Assertiveness Schedule with psychiatric population. *Behavior Therapy, 8,* 393–397.

Becker, R. E., & Heimberg, R. G. (1988). Assessment of social skills. In A. S. Bellack and M. Hersen (Eds.), *Behavioral assessment: A practical handbook* (pp. 365–395). New York: Pergamon.

RATHUS ASSERTIVENESS
SCHEDULE

Directions: Indicate how characteristic or descriptive each of the following statements is of you by using the code given below.

+3 very characteristic of me, extremely descriptive
+2 rather characteristic of me, quite descriptive
+1 somewhat characteristic of me, slightly descriptive
−1 somewhat uncharacteristic of me, slightly nondescriptive
−2 rather uncharacteristic of me, quite nondescriptive
−3 very uncharacteristic of me, extremely nondescriptive

_____ 1. Most people seem to be more aggressive and assertive than I am.*

_____ 2. *I have hesitated to make or accept dates because of "shyness."*

_____ 3. *When the food served at a restaurant is not done to my satisfaction, I complain about it to the waiter or waitress.*

_____ 4. *I am careful to avoid hurting other people's feelings, even when I feel that I have been injured.*

_____ 5. If a salesman has gone to considerable trouble to show me merchandise which is not quite suitable, I have a difficult time in saying "No."*

_____ 6. *When I am asked to do something, I insist upon knowing why.*

_____ 7. There are times when I look for a good, vigorous argument.

_____ 8. I strive to get ahead as well as most people in my position.

_____ 9. *To be honest, people often take advantage of me.*

_____ 10. I enjoy starting conversations with new acquaintances and strangers.

_____ 11. *I often don't know what to say to attractive persons of the opposite sex.*

_____ 12. *I will hesitate to make phone calls to business establishments and institutions.*

_____ 13. *I would rather apply for a job or for admission to a college by writing letters than by going through with personal interviews.*

_____ 14. *I find it embarrassing to return merchandise.*

_____ 15. If a close and respected relative were annoying me, I would smother my feelings rather than express my annoyance.*

_____ 16. *I have avoided asking questions for fear of sounding stupid.*

_____ 17. *During an argument I am sometimes afraid that I will get so upset that I will shake all over.*

_____ 18. If a famed and respected lecturer makes a statement which I think is incorrect, I will have the audience hear my point of view as well.

_____ 19. *I avoid arguing over prices with clerks and salesmen.*

_____ 20. When I have done something important or worthwhile, I manage to let others know about it.

_____ 21. I am open and frank about my feelings.

_____ 22. *If someone has been spreading false and bad stories about me, I see him (her) as soon as possible to "have a talk" about it.*

_____ 23. *I often have a hard time saying "No."*

_____ 24. *I tend to bottle up my emotions rather than make a scene.*

_____ 25. *I complain about poor service in a restaurant and elsewhere.*

_____ 26. When I am given a compliment, I sometimes just don't know what to say.*

_____ 27. If a couple near me in a theatre or at a lecture were conversing rather loudly, I would ask them to be quiet or to take their conversation elsewhere.

_____ 28. *Anyone attempting to push ahead of me in a line is in for a good battle.*

_____ 29. *I am quick to express an opinion.*

_____ 30. *There are times when I just can't say anything.**

Appendix E
Social Interaction Schedule (SIS)

This Schedule is suitable for evaluating the social skills of psychiatric patients with severe and disabling disorders in living environments; that is, in inpatient units, transitional homes or halfway houses, board-and-care homes, or day hospitals. By means of direct behavioral observation, the problems of obtaining an accurate assessment of social skills by patient not verbally articulate or perceptive can be overcome.

OBJECTIVES & PURPOSES

The purpose of the SIS is twofold:

1. It ensures that all patients, clients, or residents will have frequent contacts with a variety of staff who may help them practice their conversational skills; and
2. It provides an ongoing assessment of each patient's interpersonal behavior that can be used to evaluate change and improvement as well as to pinpoint social skills deficits requiring training or other therapeutic intervention.

The SIS has the added advantage of permitting evaluation of interpersonal behaviors in two different types of situations—during relatively unstructured time on the unit; and in one-to-one conversation with a staff member. The SIS provides data that are relevant to treatment planning, evaluation of progress and discharge readiness, and prediction of future hospital or community adjustment.

SIS Procedure

The data sheet is divided into two categories: Behavioral Observation of Social Interaction and Conversational Behavior. The SIS can be administered as frequently as staff availability and patient scheduling permit but four times daily is a minimum for reliable sources. The exact times for starting a set of observations is determined in advance and marked on the data recording sheet.

Behavioral Observation of Social Interaction

At the designated times for observation, walk through the unit, ward, or residential care home systematically. Note each patient's "Activity" and "Inappropriate Characteristics" as you go. You should record the patient's behavior at the moment you see him or her as if you only had a "snapshot" to observe. If any patient is not observed on the unit at this time, note it on the data sheet by writing "not observed" throughout the "Activity" and "Inappropriate Characteristics" blanks under his or her name.

Conversational Behavior

After completing the Behavioral Observation, initiate a conversation with each patient in the order in which their names appear on the data sheet. Approach each patient with an active curiosity about the person and a determination to find out more about them through an exchange of pleasantries, information, opinions, or feelings. To be able to make a rating on the patient's conversational skills on the data sheet, you will have to generate some two-way conversation. This will be a challenge to your social and therapeutic abilities. Here are some pointers that may help you develop spontaneous and interesting conversations:

1. Search your mind for at least two interesting, stimulating, or exciting things that have happened to you recently, which the patients might like to hear and might identify with. Starting a conversation by offering some "free information" about yourself may get the patient's response flowing.
2. Things you've read in books, magazines, newspapers or seen on TV are all excellent springboards to conversations. Current events are excellent conversation starters and offer a "bonus" in our SIS since most patients do not keep in touch with the outside world.
3. Make an effort to learn something interesting or important about the patient's life. See if you can discover things or accomplishments of which he or she is proud. Try to elicit problems or feelings that the patient may have difficulty sharing at more public times. This will give the entire team a better picture of what the patient's concerns are as well as giving you material for rating conversational skill.

4. Nonverbal contact can help expedite conversation. Position yourself so you can make good eye contact, be close physically, and even touch the patient. Every time you pat a patient on the arm or shoulder, you are sending a message such as "I like you," "I agree with what you are saying," "You've done well," or "All is well, don't worry." The power of touching can help loosen conversation by gaining attention and provide acknowledgment. A smiling facial expression, leaning toward the patient, and an open body posture are all nonverbal cues that "invite" conversation.

5. Especially for shy, withdrawn, or suspicious patients, going to a private area (bedroom, office) may loosen up the flow of conversation by making the patient more comfortable. For resistant patients, the offer of a cigarette or cup of coffee may help to establish the proper mood for conversation. But this should be brought up with team members.

6. Ask open-ended questions. For instance, instead of asking "Did you like that TV show?" ask "What did you think of that TV show?" The former close-ended question required a brief "yes" or "no" response, while the open-ended question potentially will lead to a more detailed, lengthier response.

Attempt to maintain the conversation for at least three minutes but not longer than five minutes.

This may be difficult because of the patient's delusional speech or social isolation. When the former occurs, reiterate your initial topic after briefly acknowledging the delusional segment. After the next delusional statement, inform the patient that you refuse to discuss that matter. Ignore all subsequent, delusional statements. Make sure the patient has eye contact with you by positioning yourself in his or her direct line of vision. This is especially helpful for distractable or hallucinating patients.

Such a sense of purpose may be even more important when talking to withdrawn patients. Be sure not to reinforce their unwillingness to interact by letting them "off the hook." Instead, continue to ask them questions and let them know that the best way to "get rid of you" is to respond to you. This follows the principle of negative reinforcement, where the "escape" response (in this case, the patient's verbalization) is reinforced by the termination of an aversive stimulus (i.e., your badgering).

After the conversation, rate each of the behaviors listed in the Social Interaction (Conversational Behavior) section of the data sheet on the 1–3 scale. If any inappropriate characteristics were observed during the interaction, check the appropriate box(es).

DEFINITIONS AND CRITERIA FOR MAKING RATINGS WITH THE SOCIAL INTERACTION SCHEDULE

Behavioral Observation

A. *Activity.* Activity can be recorded as either isolate or interactive. These categories are mutually exclusive, that is, every resident will fall into one and only one category.

ISOLATE: Isolate behaviors are those behaviors that a patient engages in by him- or herself. The behaviors in this category are unrelated to physical proximity or eye contact with other patients. For example, there may be two patients sitting next to each other and one of them may be talking to him- or herself, but unless it is evident that the second patient is attending to this verbalization, both patients will be regarded as engaging in isolate behavior. Isolate behavior can be divided into active and inactive categories.

1. *Active.* This category includes activities engaged in by only one patient. Examples include watching TV (eyes open and head oriented directly toward the TV), reading, writing, listening to music (singing along or moving in rhythm with the music, not merely being present while music is playing), playing solitary games, performing work, exercising, grooming, or smoking.

   If the patient is walking or running without simultaneously engaging in another behavior (isolate or active), continue to observe until it can be determined whether or not the movement is goal directed. If it is goal directed, score it as active. Examples of goal-directed walking/ running include behaviors such as going to the ping pong table to begin or watch a game, walking to a meal, walking to another person to begin an interaction. If it cannot be determined that the walking is goal directed after 10 seconds of observation, score it inactive.

2. *Inactive.* This category covers those patients who do not appear to be engaged in any of the behaviors previously defined as isolate active, such as, residents who are lying down, staring into space, and pacing, standing, sitting without doing anything else, talking to self, stripping, screaming, and other nongoal directed behaviors.

INTERACTIVE: Two patients or a patient and staff must be clearly participating in a joint activity to be scored in this category. Interactive behavior can be of a negative or positive nature.

1. *Positive.* At least two or more people must be engaged in an appropri-

ate activity—that is, behavior actively performed in the right strength and intensity for the time, place, or working constructively with at least one other individual. This includes talking, listening, playing, or working constructively with another individual. If one patient is grooming another patient or being groomed (e.g., tying shoes, combing hair), score it in this category. Arguing or disagreeing in a conversational tone should also be scored in this category.

2. *Negative.* This category includes activities that are clinically inappropriate—that is, behaviors whose strength, intensity, or content are maladaptive regardless of time, place, or circumstance, or maladaptive due to infringement on the rights of others. This category includes screaming, hitting, kicking, grabbing an object from another patient, pulling hair, and other aggressive behaviors, as well as inappropriate sexual behaviors. Any mutual bizarre activity (i.e., bizarre verbal interaction or self-stimulation) is considered negative interaction. Insults and loud arguing should be scored in this category.

If behaviors in two or more of the Activity categories are observed in the same brief observation interval, use the following priority rules to determine which one to score.

a. If behaviors in two or more of the Activity categories are observed in the brief observation interval, always score the category of the FIRST behavior observed. For example, if a positive interaction is observed and then the patient engages in isolate behavior, score only the positive interaction.

b. If interactive (positive or negative) and isolate (active or inactive) behaviors occur simultaneously during the brief observation interval, score only the interactive behavior.

c. If positive AND negative interactions occur simultaneously during the brief observation interval, score only the positive interaction.

d. If active and inactive isolate behaviors occur simultaneously during the same observation interval, score only the active behavior.

B. Inappropriate Patient Characteristics. (These categories are NOT mutually exclusive)

1. *Inappropriate Dress/Grooming* (Score if any of the following are observed):
   a. Patients without shoes. Slippers and sandals with or without socks or stockings will be considered a type of shoe, but socks or stockings alone will not.
   b. Patients with torn, dirty, excessively wrinkled, or sloppy clothing. "Dirty" refers to visual appearance and should not be evaluated

on the basis of odor. Score male patients without shirts in this category. "Sloppy" clothing would include such things as shirttails out, unless the shirt is designed to be worn out, shirt unbuttoned or buttoned incorrectly, extremely disheveled clothing, dress falling off shoulders, clothes worn inside out, pants unzipped or with broken zipper, and shoes untied.

c. Patients inappropriately dressed. This category includes bizarre dress as well as wearing clothes that are inappropriate for the temperature, setting, or time of day. Some examples of inappropriate dress are: Wearing a winter coat in the summer; wearing two shirts at the same time; wearing only underwear or pajamas in the afternoon; wearing excessive or bizarre make-up; and wearing hospital gowns. Do not attempt to determine whether or not the patient had a choice in his or her clothing selection. Simply score the patient's appearance as you observe it.

d. Inappropriate grooming. Dirt or food apparent on any part of body or clothing, hair disarrayed or obviously dirty, any part of shirttail not tucked in pants (shirts without tails should be considered inappropriately worn only if they are partially tucked in), any buttons (except collar area), snaps, zippers, laces undone, wearing bizarre make-up.

2. *On Bed, Couch, Floor* Patients on the floor. This includes those patients who have any part of their bodies except their feet in contact with the floor, or the majority of their body weight being supported by a bed or couch including those sitting upright.

3. *Talking to Self* This category includes those residents who are talking or mumbling with no apparent listener. The individual talks, makes meaningless vocalizations, or moves lips as if talking, at any time during the observation, in the absence of another who is identifiable as the intended recipient of a communication. Do not record for reading aloud, single exclamations in response to an appropriate apparent, stimulus or appropriate reactions to athletic events and shows on TV or radio.

4. *Facial Movement* Apparently involuntary wormlike wiggle of tongue, darting tongue, lateral jaw movement, rapid blinking, tremor of facial muscles, or grimacing.

5. *Repetitive and Stereotypic Body Movements* The individual (1) repeatedly moves any part of the body, continually throughout the observation, or (2) makes peculiar or bizarre gesture or other movement at any time during the observation. *Do not record for adaptive repetitive* movements such as those involved in walking, brushing teeth, combing hair, chewing gum, or eating. Rocking (not in rocking chair), repetitive hand or finger movements, repetitive self-touching such as hair pet-

ting and hand wringing, shuffling gait, rigidity of movement (i.e., hands and arms do not move in concert with legs when walking/running), gross muscle tremor.

6. *Pacing* The individual walks alone without apparent destination throughout the entire observation and the period immediately before the observation. Lack of apparent destination must be indicated by (1) walking directly toward a blank wall or "dead end" corridor, or (2) walking in an identifiable pattern such as circles or back and forth.

7. *Awake/Asleep* This category describes whether the patient is awake or asleep during the observation. Determine by the eyes—if you cannot see the eyes determine by the activity. Record only one code in this category.

   a. *Awake*. Record if the patient's eyes are open any time during the observation. If the eyes cannot be observed, record when the individual is engaged in some activity for which the eyes would ordinarily be open. Examples: squinting, one eye open, writing at desk with face not visible, leaning against wall with hand shading eyes.

   b. *Asleep*. Record if the patient's eyes are closed throughout the entire observation (unless it is clearly evident that the patient is engaged in an activity that is physically incompatible with sleep). If it is impossible to determine whether the eyes are open or closed, check this code when the individual is *not* engaged in some activity for which the eyes would ordinarily be open. Examples: napping while sitting in a chair, lying on couch with eyes closed, sitting motionless with head resting on arm or table so that face is not visible, lying motionless on bed with back to observer.

CONVERSATIONAL BEHAVIOR

A. *Eye Contact*
   1 = No or very little eye contact; excessive staring
   2 = Some avoidance of eye contact; some staring
   3 = Appropriate eye contact during the interaction

B. *Amount of Speech*
   1 = No or very little response to questions; telegraphic speech; rambling on and on, dwelling on the same subject for most of the conversation
   2 = Minimum amount of speech necessary to participate in conversation; speaking a little too much on one subject
   3 = OK; uses enough speech for one to totally understand the topic; gives complete answers to questions and volunteers additional information when appropriate

C. *Rate of Speech*

1 = So slow that speech is not understandable; speech is too fast to be understood

2 = Understandable, but obviously too fast or slow

3 = OK

D. *Voice Volume*

1 = Very soft/inaudible; very loud/screaming for no apparent reason

2 = Soft/barely audible; loud, over-normal volume for no apparent reason

3 = OK—easily audible at a distance of 3 feet

E. *Voice Inflection*

1 = Flat, monotone, no inflection; excessive, overly forceful inflection

2 = Infrequent or inappropriate inflection; moderate frequency of overly forceful inflection

3 = OK; uses appropriate inflection and inflection appropriate to content of speech

F. *Speech Intelligibility* (Coherence)

1 = Very poor; speech is obscured by distorted grammar, lack of logical connection between one part of a sentence and another or between sentences

2 = Speech is generally understandable, but frequent words or phrases not clear

3 = OK; speech is clear and understandable; only occasional words or phrases are unintelligible

G. *Speech Appropriateness* (Rationality and Relevance)

1 = Very poor; delusional speech and/or unrelated speech for conversation; ignores speech of other person. Sudden irrelevancies; grossly pedantic phrases and answering off the point; long pauses between words

2 = Minimal delusional and/or unrelated speech to flow of conversation; minimal wandering off topic

3 = OK; asks and answers questions at appropriate times during the conversation; does not wander off topic or interrupt; discusses topics generally considered appropriate for social interaction among acquaintances and friends

Social Interaction Schedule (SIS) Data Sheet

Patient _____   Date _____

	TIME OF OBSERVATION OR RATING					
BEHAVIORAL OBSERVATION OF SOCIAL INTERACTION (Check only 1)						
•Isolate Active						
•Isolate Inactive						
•Interaction Positive						
•Interaction Negative						
•Inappropriate Behaviors						
(Check only 1)						
•Awake						
•Asleep						
(Check all that apply)						
•Inappropriate Dress/Grooming						
•Talking to Self						
•On Bed, Couch, or Floor						
•Facial						
•Repetitive Stereotypic Movements						
•Pacing						

TIME OF OBSERVATION OR RATING

CONVERSATIONAL BEHAVIORS (Use 0-2-3 ratings)						
•Eye Contact						
•Amount of Speech						
•Rate and Fluency of Speech						
•Voice Volume						
•Voice Tone						
•Coherence						
•Rationality of Discourse						

Appendix F
Social Skills Distress Scale

This Scale is typical of many target complaint scales that capitalize on the fact that patients can often describe the subjective distress they experience in social situations with consistency and reliability. To use this Scale, the patient is helped to articulate the social discomfort or anxiety experienced in certain social situations using his or her own words. At each subsequent social skills training session, the patient is asked to repeatedly rate the severity of the situationally linked distress, thereby providing an opportunity to monitor the impact of training. Patients should be cautioned that changes in overt social skills usually precede improvements in subjective discomfort, often by weeks or months. The lag between behavioral skill development and feelings and attitudes is a normal and expected part of the learning process. Repeated practice of skills in real-life situations eventually yields greater social comfort and confidence.

Name _____

Complaint _____

_____

In general, how much has this problem or complaint bothered you in the past week?
Place an 'X' in the box below that best estimates your feelings.

	Date:	Date:	Date:	Date:
Couldn't be worse				
Very much				
Pretty much				
A little				
Not at all				

Appendix G
Progress Notes for Social Skills Training

MEDICAL RECORD	PROGRESS NOTES
Date	
	RMS Successful Living Group
	PROGRAM IN SOCIAL & INDEPENDENT LIVING SKILLS
	Long-Term Goals:
	Past Homework:
	Completed: Yes–No
	Short-Term Goals:
	Interpersonal Situation Rehearsed:
	Behavioral Deficits:
	Homework Assigned:
	Therapist: Extension:

(Continue on reverse side)

PATIENT'S IDENTIFICATION   CASE NO.   WARD NO.

PROGRESS NOTES

Social Skills Training Record

Name _____   Date _____

Goals: _____
_____
_____
_____

Rating:
1—Work needed
2—Improved
3—Good

Behavior Components: Trials

	Date											
Body Language													
Eye Contact													
Gestures—Descriptive —Emphatic													
Posture													
Facial Expression													

Paralinguistic Elements

Volume											
Tone											
Duration											
Fluency											
Modulation											
Latency											

Content

Appropriate to Situation											
Attentive & Receptive											
Reinforcing to Others											
Problem Solving											
Articulate											

Social Skills Training Record Sheet

Name _____ Date _____

Date	Eye Contact	Gestures	Facial Expression	Posture	Voice Tone & Loudness	Speech Fluency	Speech Content	In-Session Practice	Behavioral Assignment	Date Assignment Completed	Date Skill Generalized

Behavioral Goals

1.

2.

3.

4.

5.

6.

230

Annotated Bibliography

CONCEPTUAL FOUNDATIONS: STRESS-VULNERABILITY-COPING IN MENTAL DISORDERS

Argyle, M. (1967). *The psychology of interpersonal behavior*. Harmondsworth: Penguin.

Casey, P. R., Tyrer, P. J., & Platt, S. T. (1985). The relationship between social functioning and psychiatric symptomatology in primary care. *Social Psychiatry, 20,* 5–9.

Ciompi, L. (1987). Toward a coherent multidimensional understanding and therapy of schizophrenia: Converging new concepts. In J. S. Strauss, W. Boker, & H. D. Brenner (Eds.), *Psychosocial treatment of schizophrenia*. Toronto: Hans Huber.

Liberman, R. P., Jacobs, H. E., Boone, S. E., Foy, D. W., Donohoe, C. P., Falloon, I. R. H., Blackwell, G., & Wallace, C. J. (1987). Skills training for the community adaptation of schizophrenics. In J. Strauss, W. Boker, & H. D. Brenner (Eds.), *Psychosocial treatment of schizophrenia*. Toronto: Hans Huber.

Liberman, R. P., & Mueser, K. T. (1988). Psychosocial treatment of schizophrenia. In S. Kaplan & B. J. Sadock (Eds.), *Comprehensive textbook of psychiatry/V*. Baltimore: Wilkins & Williams.

Nuechterlein, K. H., & Dawson, M. E. (1984). A heuristic vulnerability/stress model of schizophrenic episodes. *Schizophrenia Bulletin, 10,* 300–312.

Sylph, J. A., Ross, H. E., & Kedward, H. B. (1978). Social disability in chronic psychiatric patients. *American Journal of Psychiatry, 134,* 1391–1394.

Zubin, J., & Spring, B. (1977). Vulnerability: A new view of schizophrenia. *Journal of Abnormal Psychology, 86,* 103–123.

HISTORICAL DEVELOPMENT OF SOCIAL SKILLS TRAINING

Alberti, R. E., & Emmons, M. L. (1974). *Your perfect right*. San Luis Obispo, CA: Impact Press.

Bandura, A. (1969). *Principles of behavior modification*. New York: Holt, Rinehart and Winston.

Lazarus, A. A. (1966). Behavior rehearsal vs. nondirective therapy vs. advice in effecting behavior change. *Behaviour Research and Therapy, 4,* 209–212.

Salter, A. (1949). *Conditioned reflex therapy*. New York: Farrar, Strauss.

Skinner, B. F. (1938). *The behavior of organisms: An experimental analysis*. New York: Appleton-Century-Crofts.

Wolpe, J. (1958). *Psychotherapy by reciprocal inhibition*. Stanford, CA: Stanford University Press.

Wolpe, J., & Lazarus, A. A. (1966). *Behavior therapy techniques*. New York: Pergamon Press.

ASSESSMENT OF SOCIAL SKILLS

Arkowitz, H. (1988). Assessment of social skills. In M. Hersen & A. S. Bellack (Eds.), *Behavioral assessment: A practical handbook* (2nd ed.). Oxford: Pergamon Press.

Bellack, A. S. (1979). A critical appraisal of strategies for assessing social skill. *Behavior Assessment, 1*, 157–176.

Bellack, A. S. (1983). Recurrent problems in the behavioral assessment of social skill. *Behaviour Research and Therapy, 21*, 29–42.

Bellack, A. S., Hersen, M., & Lamparski, D. (1979). Roleplay tests for assessing social skills: Are they valid? Are they useful? *Journal of Consulting and Clinical Psychology, 47*, 335–342.

Connor, J., Dann, L., & Twentyman, C. (1982). A self-report measure of assertiveness in young adolescents. *Journal of Clinical Psychology, 38*, 101–106.

Curran, J. P. (1979). Pandora's Box reopened? The assessment of social skills. *Journal of Behavioral Assessment, 1*, 55–72.

Curran, J. P. (1982). A procedure for the assessment of social skills: The simulated social interaction test. In J. P. Curran & P. M. Monti (Eds.), *Social skills training: A practical handbook for assessment and treatment*. New York: Guilford.

Dow, M. G., Glaser, S. R., & Biglan, A. B. (1981). The relevance of specific conversational behaviors to ratings of social skill: An experimental analysis. *Journal of Behavioral Assessment, 3*, 233–242.

Eisler, R. M., Miller, P. M., & Hersen, M. (1973). Components of assertive behavior. *Journal of Clinical Psychology, 29*, 295–299.

Hersen, M., Eisler, R. M., & Miller, P. M. (1973). Development of assertive responses: Clinical, measurement, and research consideration. *Behaviour Research and Therapy, 11*, 505–521.

Laws, D. R., & Serber, M. (1974). Measurement and evaluation of Assertive Training with sexual offenders. In R. E. Hosford & S. Moss (Eds.), *The crumbling walls: Treatment and counseling of the youthful offender*. Champaign, IL: University of Illinois Press.

Liberman, R. P. (1982). Assessment of social skills. *Schizophrenia Bulletin, 8*, 62–82.

Rathus, S. A. (1973). A 30-item schedule for assessing assertive behavior. *Behavior Therapy, 4*, 398–406.

Wallace, C. J. (1986). Functional assessment in rehabilitation. *Schizophrenia Bulletin, 12*, 604–630.

CLINICAL MANUALS
AND HANDBOOKS

Becker, R. E., Heimberg, R. G., & Bellack, A. S. (1987). *Social skills training treatment for depression*. New York: Pergamon Press.

Eisler, R. M., & Frederiksen, L. W. (1980). *Perfecting social skills: A guide to interpersonal behavior development*. New York: Plenum.

Ellis, R., & Wittington, D. (1981). *A guide to social skills training*. London: Croom Helm.

Goldstein, A. P. (1973). *Structured learning therapy*. New York: Academic Press.

Goldstein, A. P. (in press). *Psychological skill training: The structured learning approach*. New York: Pergamon Press.

Goldstein, A. P., Sprafkin, R. P., & Gershaw, N. J. (1976). *Skill training for community living: Applying structured learning therapy*. New York: Pergamon Press.

Goldstein, A. P., Sprafkin, R. P., Gershaw, N. J., & Klein, P. (1980). *Skillstreaming the adolescent*. Champaign, IL: Research Press.

Hargie, O., & McCartan, P. J. (1986). *Social skills and psychiatric nursing*. London: Croom Helm.

Kelly, J. A. (1982). *Social skills training: A practical guide for interventions*. New York: Springer.

Lange, A. J., & Jakubowski, P. (1976). *Responsible assertive behavior*. Champaign, IL: Research Press.

Liberman, R. P., King, K. W., DeRisi, W. J., & McCann, M. (1975). *Personal effectiveness: Guiding people to assert themselves and improve their social skills*. (Therapist Manual, Client's Brochure, Training Guide, & Demonstration Video). Champaign, IL: Research Press. (Available from Psychiatric Rehabilitation Consultants, Camarillo–UCLA Research Center, Box A, Camarillo, CA 93011)

Liberman, R. P., & Associates (1986–89). *Modules for training social and independent living skills* (Trainer's Manual, Patient's Workbook, Demonstration Video). (Available from Psychiatric Rehabilitation Consultants, Camarillo–UCLA Research Center, Box A, Camarillo, CA 93011)

    Medication Management

    Symptom Management

    Recreation for Leisure

    Self-care & Grooming

    Conversation Skills

Trower, P., Bryant, B., & Argyle, M. (1978). *Social skills and mental health*. Pittsburgh: University of Pittsburgh Press.

Wilkinson, J., & Canter, S. (1982). *Social skills training manual*. New York: John Wiley.

SCHOLARLY BOOKS

Bellack, A. S., & Hersen, M. (Eds.). (1979). *Research and practice in social skills training*. New York: Plenum.

Curran, J. P., & Monti, P. M. (Eds.). (1982). *Social skills training*. New York: Guilford.

Hollin, C. R., & Trower, P. (Eds.). (1986). *Handbook of social skills training* (Vols. I–II). New York: Pergamon Press.

L'Abate, L., & Milan, M. A. (Eds.). (1985). *Handbook of social skills training and research*. New York: John Wiley.

Spence, S., & Shepherd, G. (Eds.). (1983). *Developments in social skills training*. London: Academic Press.

Trower, P. (Ed.). (1984). *Radical approaches to social skills training*. London: Croom Helm.

Trower, P., Bryant, B., & Argyle, M. (1978). *Social skills and mental health*. Pittsburgh: University of Pittsburgh Press.

OVERVIEWS OF
SOCIAL SKILLS TRAINING

Bellack, A. S., & Mueser, K. T. (1986). A comprehensive treatment program for schizophrenia and chronic mental illness. *Community Mental Health Journal, 22*, 175–189.

Brady, J. P. (1984a). Social skills training for psychiatric patients. I: Concepts, methods, and clinical results. *American Journal of Psychiatry, 141*, 333–340.

Brady, J. P. (1984b). Social skills training for psychiatric patients. II: Clinical outcome studies. *American Journal of Psychiatry, 141*, 491–498.

Fensterheim, H. (1972). Assertive Training in groups. In C. J. Sager & H. S. Kaplan (Eds.), *Progress in group and family therapy*. New York: Brunner/Mazel.

Foy, D. W., Wallace, C. J., & Liberman, R. P. (1983). Advances in social skills training for chronic mental patients. In K. D. Craig & M. J. McMahon (Eds.), *Advances in clinical behavior therapy*. New York: Brunner/Mazel.

Hersen, M., & Bellack, A. S. (1976). Social skills training for chronic psychiatric patients: Rationale, research findings, and future directions. *Comprehensive Psychiatry, 17*, 559–580.

Hersen, M., & Eisler, P. M. (1976). Social skills training. In W. E. Craighead, A. E. Kazdin, & M. J. Mahoney (Eds.), *Behavior modification: Principles, issues, and applications*. Boston: Houghton-Mifflin.

Hierholzer, R. W., & Liberman, R. P. (1986). Successful living: A social skills and problem-solving group for the chronic mentally ill. *Hospital and Community Psychiatry, 37*, 913–918.

Hollin, C. R., & Trower, P. (1988). Development and applications of social skills training: A review and critique. In M. Hersen, R. M. Eisler, & P. M. Miller (Eds.), *Progress in behavior modification* (Vol. 22). Newbury Park, CA: Sage.

Liberman, R. P., Falloon, I. R. H., & Wallace, C. J. (1984). Drug psychosocial interventions in the treatment of schizophrenia. In M. Mirabi (Ed.), *The chronically mentally ill: Research and services* (pp. 175–212). New York: SP Medical & Scientific Books.

Liberman, R. P., Massel, H. K., Mosk, M. D., & Wong, S. E. (1985). Social skills training for chronic mental patients. *Hospital and Community Psychiatry, 36*, 396–403.

Liberman, R. P., Mueser, K. T., Wallace, C. J., Jacobs, H. E., Eckman, T., & Massel, H. K. (1986). Training skills to the psychiatrically disabled: Learning coping and competence. *Schizophrenia Bulletin, 12*, 631–647.

Liberman, R. P., Nuechterlein, K. H., & Wallace, C. J. (1982). Social skills training and the nature of schizophrenia. In J. P. Curran & P. M. Monti (Eds.), *Social skills training: A practical handbook for assessment and treatment* (pp. 5–56). New York: Guilford.

McFall, R. M. (1982). A review and reformulation of the concept of social skills. *Behavioral Assessment, 4*, 1–33.

Monti, P. M., & Kolko, D. J. (1985). A review and programmatic model of group social skills training for psychiatric patients. In D. Upper & S. M. Ross (Eds.), *Handbook of behavioral group therapy*. New York: Plenum.

Morrison, R. L., & Bellack, A. S. (1985). Social skills training. In A. S. Bellack (Ed.), *Schizophrenia: Treatment, management, and rehabilitation* (pp. 247–279). Orlando, FL: Grune & Stratton.

Twentyman, G. T., & Zimmering, R. T. (1979). Behavioral training of social skills: A critical review. In M. Hersen, R. M. Eisler, & P. M. Miller (Eds.), *Progress in behavior modification* (Vol. 7). New York: Academic Press.

Wallace, C. J., & Boone, S. E. (1984). Cognitive factors in the social skills of schizophrenic patients: Implications for treatment. In W. D. Spaulding & J. K. Cole (Eds.), *Theories of schizophrenia and psychosis, Nebraska Symposium on Motivation* (Vol. 31). Lincoln: University of Nebraska Press.

Wallace, C. J., Boone, S. E., Donahoe, C. P., & Foy, D. W. (1985). Psychosocial rehabilitation for the chronic mentally disabled: Social and independent living skills training. In D. Barlow (Ed.), *Behavioral treatment of adult disorders*. New York: Guilford.

Wallace, C. J., Nelson, C. J., Liberman, R. P., Aitchison, R. A., Lukoff, D., Elder, J. P., & Ferris, C. (1980). A review and critique of social skills training with schizophrenic patients. *Schizophrenia Bulletin, 6*, 42–63.

Wixted, J. T., Morrison, R. L., & Bellack, A. S. (1988). Social skills training in the treatment of negative symptoms. *International Journal of Mental Health, 17*, 3–21.

TREATMENT OUTCOME STUDIES
WITH PSYCHIATRIC PATIENTS

Bellack, A. S., Hersen, M., & Turner, S. M. (1976). Generalization effects of social skills training with chronic schizophrenics: An experimental analysis. *Behaviour Research and Therapy, 14*, 391–398.

Bellack, A. S., Turner, S. M., Hersen, M., & Luber, R. F. (1984). An examination of the efficacy of social skills training for chronic schizophrenic patients. *Hospital and Community Psychiatry, 35*, 1023–1028.

Bennett, P. S., & Maley, R. G. (1973). Modification of interactive behaviors in chronic mental patients. *Journal of Applied Behavior Analysis, 6*, 609–620.

Brown, M. A., & Munford, A. M. (1983). Life skills training for chronic schizophrenia. *Journal of Nervous and Mental Disease, 171*, 466–470.

Eisler, R. M., Blanchard, E. B., Fitts, H., & Williams, J. G. (1978). Social skill training with and without modeling for schizophrenic and non-psychotic hospitalized psychiatric patients. *Behavior Modification, 2*, 147–172.

Falloon, I. R. H., Lindley, D. P., McDonald, R., & Marks, I. M. (1977). Social skills training of outpatient groups: A controlled study of rehearsal and homework. *British Journal of Psychiatry, 131*, 599–609.

Fichter, M., Wallace, C. J., Liberman, R. P., & Davis, J. R. (1976). Improving social interaction in a chronic psychotic using "nagging" (discriminated avoidance): Experimental analysis and generalization. *Journal of Applied Behavior Analysis, 9*, 377–386.

Foxx, R. M., McMorrow, M. J., Bittle, R. G., & Fenlon, S. J. (1985). Teaching social skills to psychiatric inpatients. *Behaviour Research and Therapy, 23*, 531–537.

Goldsmith, J. B., & McFall, R. M. (1975). Development and evaluation of an interpersonal skill-training program for psychiatric inpatients. *Journal of Abnormal Psychology, 84*, 51–58.

Goldstein, A. P., Marten, J., Hubben, J., Van Belle, H. A., Schaaf, W., Wierema, H., & Goedhart, A. (1973). The use of modeling to increase independent behavior. *Behaviour Research and Therapy, 11*, 31–42.

Gutride, M. E., Goldstein, A. P., & Hunter, G. F. (1973). The use of modeling and roleplaying to increase social interactions among asocial psychiatric patients. *Journal of Consulting and Clinical Psychology, 40*, 408–415.

Hersen, M., & Bellack, A. S. (1976). A multiple-baseline analysis of social-skills training in chronic schizophrenics. *Journal of Applied Behavior Analysis, 9*, 239–245.

Hersen, M., Eisler, R. M., & Miller, P. M. (1974). An experimental analysis of generalization in Assertive Training. *Behaviour Research and Therapy, 12*, 295–310.

Hersen, M., Eisler, R. M., Miller, P. M., Johnson, M. B., & Pinkston, S. G. (1973). Effects of practice, instructions and modeling on components of assertive behavior. *Behaviour Research and Therapy, 11*, 443–451.

Hogarty, G. E., Anderson, C. M., Reiss, D. J., Kornblith, S. J., Greenwald, D. P., Javna, C. D., & Madonia, M. J. (1986). Family psycho-education, social skills training and maintenance chemotherapy in the aftercare of schizophrenia: 1. One-year effects of a controlled study on relapse and expressed emotion. *Archives of General Psychiatry, 43*, 633–642.

King, L. W., Liberman, R. P., Roberts, J., & Bryan, E. (1977). Personal effectiveness: A structured therapy for improving social and emotional skills. *European Journal of Behavioral Analysis and Modification, 2*, 82–91.

Liberman, R. P., Lillie, F. J., Falloon, I. R. H., Harpin, E. J., Hutchinson, W., & Stouts, B. A. (1984). Social skills training for relapsing schizophrenics: An experimental analysis. *Behavior Modification, 8*, 155–179.

Liberman, R. P., Mueser, K. T., & Wallace, C. J. (1986). Social skills training for schizophrenics at risk for relapse. *American Journal of Psychiatry, 143*, 523–526.

Lindsay, W. F., & Stoffelmayr, B. E. (1982). The concept of generalization in behaviour therapy. *Behavioural Psychotherapy, 10*, 346–355.

Marzillier, J. S., Lambert, J. C., & Kellett, J. (1976). A controlled evaluation of systematic desensitisation and social skills training for chronically inadequate psychiatric patients. *Behaviour Research and Therapy, 14*, 225–229.

Monti, P. M., Curran, J. P., Coriveau, D. P., DeLancey, A. L., & Hagerman, S. M. (1980). Effects of social skills training groups and sensitivity training groups with psychiatric patients. *Journal of Consulting and Clinical Psychology, 48*, 241–248.

Wallace, C. J., & Liberman, R. P. (1985). Social skills training for patients with schizophrenia: A controlled clinical trial. *Psychiatry Research, 14*, 239–247.

Wong, S. E., Terranova, M. D., Bowen, L., Zarate, T., Massel, H. K., & Liberman, R. P. (1987). Providing independent recreational activities to reduce stereotypic vocalizations in chronic schizophrenics. *Journal of Applied Behavior Analysis, 20*, 77–81.

APPLICATION OF
SOCIAL SKILLS TRAINING
TO CLINICAL PROBLEMS

Alcohol and Drug Abuse

Botvin, G. J., Baker, E., Renick, N. L., Filazzola, A. D., & Botvin, E. M. (1984). A cognitive-behavioral approach to substance abuse prevention. *Addictive Behaviors, 9*, 137–147.

Botvin, G. J., & Willis, T. A. (1985). *Cognitive-behavioral approaches to substance abuse prevention.* (National Institute on Drug Abuse Research Monograph Series, Monograph 63, pp. 8–49). Bethesda, MD: NIDA.

Callahan, E. J., Rawson, R. A., McCleave, B., Arias, R., Glazer, M., & Liberman, R. P. (1980). The treatment of heroin addiction: Naltrexone alone and with behavior therapy. *International Journal of the Addictions, 15*, 795–807.

Callner, D. A., & Ross, S. M. (1978). The assessment and training of assertive skills with drug addicts: A preliminary study. *International Journal of the Addictions, 13*, 227–229.

Chaney, E. F., O'Leary, M. R., & Marlatt, G. A. (1978). Skill training with alcoholics. *Journal of Consulting and Clinical Psychology, 46*, 1092–1104.

Cheek, F. E., Tomarchio, T., Standen, J., & Albahary, R. S. (1973). Methadone plus—A behavior modification training program in self-control for addicts on methadone maintenance. *International Journal of the Addictions, 8*, 969–996.

Eriksen, L., Bjornstad, S., & Gotestam, K. (1986). Social skills training in groups for alcoholics: One-year treatment outcome for groups and individuals. *Addictive Behaviors, 11*, 309–329.

Foy, D. W., Miller, P. M., Eisler, R. M., & O'Toole, D. M. (1976). Social skills training to teach alcoholics to refuse drinks effectively. *Journal of Studies on Alcohol, 37*, 1340–1345.

Foy, D. W., Nunn, L. B., & Rychtarik, R. G. (1984). Broad-spectrum behavioral treatment for chronic alcoholics: Effects of training controlled drinking skills. *Journal of Consulting and Clinical Psychology, 52*, 218–230.

Hawkins, J. D., Catalano, R. F., & Wells, E. A. (1986). Measuring effects of a skills training intervention for drug abusers. *Journal of Consulting and Clinical Psychology, 54*, 661–664.

Hersen, M., Miller, P. M., & Eisler, R. M. (1973). Interactions between alcoholics and their wives: A descriptive analysis of verbal and nonverbal behavior. *Quarterly Journal of Studies on Alcohol, 34*, 516–520.

Lin, T., Bon, S., Dickinson, J., & Blume, C. (1982). Systematic development and evaluation of a social skills training program for chemical abusers. *International Journal of the Addictions, 17*, 585–596.

Miller, P. M., & Eisler, R. M. (1977). Assertive behavior of alcoholics: A descriptive analysis. *Behavior Therapy, 8*, 146–149.

Miller, P. M., Hersen, M., Eisler, R. M., & Hilsman, G. (1974). Effects of social stress on operant drinking of alcoholics and social drinkers. *Behaviour Research and Therapy, 12*, 67–72.

Monti, P. M., Abrams, D. B., Binkoff, J. A., & Zwick, W. R. (1986). Social skills training in substance abuse. In C. R. Hollin & P. Trower (Eds.), *Handbook of social skills training*, Vol. 2 (pp. 111–142). New York: Pergamon Press.

Oei, T. P. S., & Jackson, P. R. (1982). Social skills and cognitive behavioral approaches to the treatment of problem drinking. *Journal of Studies on Alcohol, 43*, 532–546.

Van Hasselt, V. B., Hersen, M., & Milliones, J. (1978). Social skills training for alcoholics and drug addicts: A review. *Addictive Behaviors, 3*, 221–233.

Watson, D. W., & Maisto, S. A. (1983). A review of the effectiveness of assertiveness training in the treatment of alcohol abusers. *Behavioral Psychotherapy, 11*, 36–49.

Anger and Aggression

Benson, B. A., Rice, C. J., & Miranti, S. V. (1986). Effects of anger management training with mentally retarded adults in group treatment. *Journal of Consulting and Clinical Psychology, 54*, 728–729.

Deffenbacher, J. L., Story, D. A., Stark, R. S., Hogg, J. A., & Brandon, A. D. (1987). Cognitive-relaxation and social skills interventions in the treatment of general anger. *Journal of Counseling Psychology, 34*, 171–176.

Elder, J., Edelstein, B., & Narick, M. (1979). Adolescent psychiatric patients: Modifying aggressive behavior with social skills training. *Behavior Modification, 3*, 161–178.

Feindler, E. L., & Ecton, R. B. (1986). *Adolescent anger control*. New York: Pergamon Press.

Feindler, E. L., Ecton, R. B., Kingsley, D., & Dubey, D. R. (1986). Group anger-control training for institutionalized psychiatric male adolescents. *Behavior Therapy, 17*, 109–123.

Foy, D. W., Eisler, R. M., & Pinkston, S. (1975). Modeled assertion in a case of explosive rages. *Journal of Behavior Therapy and Experimental Psychiatry, 6*, 135–137.

Frederickson, L. W., Jenkins, J. O., Foy, D. W., & Eisler, R. M. (1976). Social skills training to modify abusive verbal outbursts in adults. *Journal of Applied Behavior Analysis, 9*, 117–127.

Goldstein, A. P., & Keller, H. (1987). *Aggressive behavior: Assessment and intervention*. New York: Pergamon Press.

Goldstein, A. P., & Pentz, M. A. (1984). Psychological skill training and the aggressive adolescent. *School Psychology Review, 13*, 311–323.

Goodwin, S., & Mahoney, M. (1975). Modification of aggression via modeling: An experimental probe. *Journal of Behavior Therapy and Experimental Psychiatry, 6*, 200–202.

Kolko, D. J., Dorsett, P., & Milan, M. (1981). A total-assessment approach in the evaluation of social-skills training: The effectiveness of an anger control program for adolescent psychiatric patients. *Behavior Assessment, 3*, 383–402.

Jamison, R. N., Lambert, E. W., & McCloud, D. J. (1985). Social skills training with hospitalized adolescents: An evaluative experiment. *Adolescence, 21*, 55–65.

Liberman, R. P., Marshall, B. D., & Burke, K. (1981). Drug and environmental interventions for aggressive psychiatric patients. In R. B. Stuart (Ed.), *Control of violence* (pp. 227–264). New York: Brunner/Mazel.

Matson, J., & Stephens, R. (1978). Increasing appropriate behavior of explosive chronic psychiatric patients with a social skills training package. *Behavior Modification, 2,* 61–76.

Moon, J. R., & Eisler, R. M. (1983). Anger control: An experimental comparison of three behavioral treatments. *Behavior Therapy, 14,* 493–505.

Novaco, R. W. (1975). *Anger control.* Lexington, MA: D. C. Heath.

Rahain, S., Lefebure, C., & Jenkins, J. O. (1980). The effects of social skills training on behavioral and cognitive components of anger management. *Journal of Behavior Therapy and Experimental Psychiatry, 11,* 3–8.

Rimm, D., Hill, G., Brown, N., & Stuart, J. (1974). Group assertion training in the treatment of inappropriate anger. *Psychological Reports, 34,* 791–798.

Wallace, C. J., Teigen, J. R., Liberman, R. P., & Baker, V. (1973). Destructive behavior treated by contingency contracts and assertive training: A case study. *Journal of Behavior Therapy and Experimental Psychiatry, 4,* 273–274.

Wong, S., Slama, K., & Liberman, R. P. (1986). Behavior analysis and therapy for aggressive psychiatric and developmentally disabled patients. In L. Roth (Ed.), *Clinical treatment of the violent person.* New York: Guilford.

Anxiety and Social Avoidance

Alstrom, J. E., Nordlund, C. L., Persson, G., Harding, M., & Ljungqvist, C. (1984). Effects of four treatment methods on social phobic patients not suitable for insight-oriented psychotherapy. *Acta Psychiatrica Scandinavica, 70,* 97–110.

Argyle, M., Trower, P. E., & Bryant, B. M. (1974). Explorations in the treatment of personality disorders and neuroses by social skills training. *British Journal of Medical Psychology, 47,* 63–72.

Cappe, R. F., & Alden, L. E. (1986). A comparison of treatment strategies for clients functionally impaired by extreme shyness and social avoidance. *Journal of Consulting and Clinical Psychology, 54,* 796–801.

Curran, J. P., Monti, P. M., Corriveau, D. P., Hay, L. R., Hagerman, S., Zwick, W. R., & Farrell, A. D. (1980). The generalizability of a procedure for assessing social skills and social anxiety in a psychiatric population. *Behavioral Assessment, 2,* 389–402.

Halford, K., & Foddy, D. M. (1982). Cognitive and social skills correlates of social anxiety. *British Journal of Clinical Psychology, 21,* 17–28.

Marshall, P. G., Keltner, A. A., & Marshall, W. L. (1981). Anxiety reduction, assertive training, and enactment of consequences. *Behavior Modification, 5,* 85–102.

Rehm, L. P., & Marston, A. R. (1968). Reduction of social anxiety through modification of self-reinforcement: An instigation therapy technique. *Journal of Consulting and Clinical Psychology, 32,* 565–574.

Stravynski, A., Grey, S., & Elie, R. (1987). Outline of the therapeutic process in social skills training and socially dysfunctional patients. *Journal of Consulting and Clinical Psychology, 55,* 224–228.

Stravynski, A., & Shahar, A. (1983). The treatment of social dysfunction in non-psychotic outpatients: A review. *Journal of Nervous and Mental Disease, 171,* 721–728.

Trower, P. (1986). Social skills training and social anxiety. In C. R. Hollin & P. Trower (Eds.), *Handbook of social skills training: Vol. 2. Clinical applications and new directions.* Oxford: Pergamon Press.

Trower, P., Yardley, K., Bryant, B., & Shaw, P. (1978). The treatment of social failure: A comparison of anxiety reduction and skills acquisition procedures in two social problems. *Behavior Modification, 2,* 41–46.

Twentyman, G. T., & McFall, R. M. (1975). Behavioral training of social skills in shy males. *Journal of Consulting and Clinical Psychology, 43,* 384–395.

Assertiveness

Alberti, R. E., & Emmons, M. L. (1974). *Your perfect right*. San Luis Obispo, CA: Impact Press.

Edwards, N. B. (1972). Assertive Training in a case of homosexual pedophilia. *Journal of Behavior Therapy and Experimental Psychiatry, 3*, 55–63.

Eisler, R. M., Hersen, M., & Miller, P. M. (1973). Effects of modeling on components of assertive behavior. *Journal of Behavior Therapy and Experimental Psychiatry, 4*, 1–6.

Eisler, R. M., Hersen, M., & Miller, P. M. (1974). Shaping components of assertive behavior with instructions and feedback. *American Journal of Psychiatry, 131*, 1344–1347.

Eisler, R. M., Hersen, M., Miller, P. M., & Blanchard, E. B. (1975). Situational determinants of assertive behaviors. *Journal of Consulting and Clinical Psychology, 43*, 330–340.

Eisler, R. M., Miller, P. M., & Hersen, M. (1973). Components of assertive behavior. *Journal of Clinical Psychology, 29*, 295–299.

Field, G. D., & Test, M. A. (1975). Group assertive training for severely disturbed patients. *Journal of Behavior Therapy and Experimental Psychiatry, 6*, 129–134.

Finch, B. E., & Wallace, C. J. (1977). Successful interpersonal skills training with schizophrenic inpatients. *Journal of Consulting and Clinical Psychology, 45*, 885–890.

Galassi, J. P., Galassi, M. D., & Litz, M. C. (1974). Assertive training in groups using video feedback. *Journal of Consulting and Clinical Psychology, 21*, 390–394.

Hammen, C. L., Jacobs, M., Mayol, A., & Cochran, S. D. (1980). Dysfunctional cognitions and the effectiveness of skills and cognitive-behavioral assertion training. *Journal of Consulting and Clinical Psychology, 48*, 685–695.

Hatzenbuehler, L., & Schroeder, H. E. (1982). Assertiveness training with outpatients: The effectiveness of skill and cognitive procedures. *Behavioral Psychotherapy, 10*, 234–252.

Hersen, M., Eisler, R. M., & Miller, P. M. (1973). Development of assertive responses: Clinical, measurement, and research considerations. *Behaviour Research and Therapy, 11*, 505–521.

Hersen, M., Eisler, R. M., & Miller, P. M. (1974). An experimental analysis of generalization in assertive training. *Behaviour Research and Therapy, 12*, 295–310.

Hersen, M., Eisler, R. M., Miller, P. M., Johnson, M. B., & Pinkston, S. G. (1973). Effects of practice, instructions and modeling on components of assertive behavior. *Behaviour Research and Therapy, 11*, 443–451.

Kelly, J. A., Frederiksen, L. W., Fitts, H., & Phillips, J. (1978). Training and generalization of commendatory assertiveness: A controlled single subject experiment. *Journal of Behavior Therapy and Experimental Psychiatry, 9*, 17–21.

Lange, A. J., & Jakubowski, P. (1976). *Responsible assertive behavior*. Champaign, IL: Research Press.

Linehan, M. M. (1979). Assertion therapy: Skill training or cognitive restructuring. *Behavior Therapy, 10*, 372–388.

McFall, R. M., & Lillesand, D. B. (1971). Behavioral rehearsal with modeling and coaching in Assertion Training. *Journal of Abnormal Psychology, 77*, 313–323.

McFall, R. M., & Marston, A. R. (1970). An experimental investigation of behavioral rehearsal in Assertive Training. *Journal of Abnormal Psychology, 76*, 295–303.

McFall, R. M., & Twentyman, C. T. (1973). Four experiments on the relative contributions of rehearsal, modeling, and coaching to assertion training. *Journal of Abnormal Psychology, 81*, 199–218.

McFall, R. M., Winnett, R. L., Bordewick, M. C., & Bornstein, P. H. (1982). Nonverbal components in the communication of assertiveness. *Behavior Modification, 6*, 121–140.

Patterson, R. (1972). Time-out and Assertive Training for a dependent child. *Behavior Therapy, 3*, 466–468.

Rathus, S. A. (1972). An experimental investigation of Assertive Training in a group setting. *Journal of Behavior Therapy and Experimental Psychiatry, 3,* 81–86.

Romano, J. M., & Bellack, A. S. (1980). Social validation of a component model of assertive behavior. *Journal of Consulting and Clinical Psychology, 48,* 478–490.

Serber, M. (1972). Teaching the nonverbal components of Assertive Training. *Journal of Behavior Therapy and Experimental Psychiatry, 3,* 1–5.

Weinman, B., Gelbart, P., Wallace, M., & Post, M. (1972). Inducing assertive behavior in chronic schizophrenics: A comparison of socioenvironmental, desensitization, and relaxation therapies. *Journal of Consulting and Clinical Psychology, 39,* 246–252.

Conversational Skill

Bradlyn, A. S., Himadi, W. G., Crimmins, D. B., Graves, K. G., & Kelly, J. A. (1983). Conversational skills training for retarded adolescents. *Behavior Therapy, 14,* 314–325.

Christoff, K. A., Scott, W. O. N., Kelly, M. L., Schlundt, D., Baer, G., & Kelly, J. A. (1985). Social skills and social problem-solving training for shy young adolescents. *Behavior Therapy, 16,* 468–477.

Dow, M. G., Glaser, S. R., & Biglan, A. B. (1981). The relevance of specific conversational behaviors to ratings of social skill: An experimental analysis. *Journal of Behavioral Assessment, 3,* 233–242.

Eckman, T. A. (1976). An educational workshop in conversational skills. In J. D. Krumboltz & C. E. Thorensen (Eds.), *Counseling methods.* New York: Holt, Rinehart and Winston.

Hargie, O. (Ed.). (1986). *Handbook of communication skills.* New York: New York University Press.

Holmes, M. R., Hansen, D. J., & St. Lawrence, J. S. (1984). Conversational skills training with aftercare patients in the community: Social validation and generalization. *Behavior Therapy, 15,* 84–100.

Kelly, J. A., Furman, W., Phillips, J., Hathorn, S., & Wilson, T. (1979). Teaching conversational skills to retarded adolescents. *Child Behavior Therapy, 1,* 85–97.

Kupke, T., Hobbs, S. A., Lavin, P. F., & Cheney, T. H. (1984). Social validation of a conversational skills training program. *Journal of Behavioral Assessment, 6,* 219–230.

Lewis, F. D., Roessler, R., Greenwood, R, & Evans, T. (1985). Conversational skill training with individuals with severe emotional disabilities. *Psychosocial Rehabilitation Journal, 8,* 49–59.

Lindsay, W. R. (1980). The training and generalization of conversation behaviours in psychiatric in-patients: A controlled study employing multiple measures across settings. *British Journal of Social and Clinical Psychology, 19,* 85–98.

Lindsay, W. R. (1982). Some normative goals for conversation training. *Behavioral Psychotherapy, 10,* 253–272.

McGee, G., Krantz, P. J., & McClannahan, L. E. (1984). Conversational skills for autistic adolescents: Teaching assertiveness in naturalistic game settings. *Journal of Autism and Developmental Disorders, 14,* 319–330.

Minkin, N., Braukmann, C. J., Minkin, B. L., Timbers, G. D., Timbers, B. J., Fixsen, D. J., Phillips, E. L., & Wolf, M. M. (1976). The social validation and training of conversational skills. *Journal of Applied Behavior Analysis, 9,* 127–139.

Plienis, A. J., Hansen, D. J., Ford, F., Smith, Jr., S., Stark, L. J., & Kelly, J. A. (1987). Behavioral small group training to improve the social skills of emotionally disordered adolescents. *Behavior Therapy, 18,* 17–32.

Praderas, K., & McDonald, M. L. (1986). Telephone conversational skills training with socially isolated, impaired nursing home residents. *Journal of Applied Behavior Analysis, 19,* 337–348.

Rubin, J. H., & Locascio, K. (1985). A model of communication skills group using structured exercises and audiovisual equipment. *International Journal of Group Psychotherapy, 35,* 569–584.

Urey, J. R., Laughlin, C. S., & Kelly, J. A. (1979). Teaching heterosocial conversational skills to male psychiatric "inpatients." *Journal of Behavior Therapy and Experimental Psychiatry, 10,* 323–328.

Wallace, C. J., & Davis, J. R. (1974). The effects of information and reinforcement on the conversational behavior of chronic psychiatric patient dyads. *Journal of Consulting and Clinical Psychology, 42,* 656–666.

Wildman, B. G., Wildman, H. E., & Kelly, J. W. (1986). Group conversational skills training and social validation with mentally retarded adults. *Applied Research in Mental Retardation, 7,* 443–458.

Depression

Bellack, A. S., Hersen, M., & Himmelhoch, J. M. (1983). A comparison of social skills training, pharmacotherapy and psychotherapy for depression. *Behaviour Research and Therapy, 21,* 101–107.

deJong, R., Treiber, R., & Gerhard, H. (1986). Effectiveness of two psychological treatments for inpatients with severe and chronic depressions. *Cognitive Therapy and Research, 10,* 645–663.

Harpin, R. E. (1981). Behavior therapy for chronically depressed patients: A clinical report. *Psychological Reports, 48,* 763–774.

Jansson, L. (1984). Social skills training for unipolar depression: A case study. *Scandinavian Journal of Behaviour Therapy, 13,* 237–241.

Lewinsohn, P. M., & Shaw, D. A. (1969). Feedback about interpersonal behavior as an agent of behavior change: A case study in the treatment of depression. *Psychotherapy and Psychosomatics, 17,* 82–88.

Libet, J., & Lewinsohn, P. M. (1973). The concept of social skills with special reference to the behavior of depressed persons. *Journal of Consulting and Clinical Psychology, 40,* 304–312.

McKnight, D. L., Nelson, R. O., Hayes, S. C., & Jarrett, R. B. (1984). Importance of treating individually assessed response classes in the amelioration of depression. *Behavior Therapy, 15,* 315–335.

Rehm, L. P., Fuchs, C. Z., Roth, D. M., Kornblith, S. J., & Romano, J. M. (1979). A comparison of self-control and assertion skills treatments of depression. *Behavior Therapy, 10,* 429–442.

Sanchez, V. C., Lewinsohn, P. M., & Larson, D. W. (1980). Assertion training: Effectiveness in the treatment of depression. *Journal of Clinical Psychology, 37,* 527–529.

Schotts, D. E., & Clum, G. A. (1987). Problem-solving skills in suicidal psychiatric patients. *Journal of Consulting and Clinical Psychology, 55,* 49–53.

Zeiss, A. M., Lewinsohn, P. M., & Munoz, R. F. (1979). Nonspecific improvement effects in depression using interpersonal skills training, pleasant activity schedule, or cognitive training. *Journal of Consulting and Clinical Psychology, 45,* 543–551.

Marital and Family Therapy

Alevizos, P. N., & Liberman, R. P. (1975). Behavioral approaches to family crisis intervention. In H. L. P. Resnick & H. Parad (Eds.), *Innovations in emergency mental health services.* Bowie, MD: Brady.

Bornstein, P. H., & Bornstein, M. T. (1985). *Marital therapy: A behavioral-communication approach*. New York: Pergamon Press.

Christensen, A., & Nies, D. C. (1980). The Spouse Observation Checklist: Empirical analysis and critique. *American Journal of Family Therapy, 8*, 69–79.

Eisler, R. M., & Hersen, M. (1973). Behavioral techniques in family-oriented crisis intervention. *Archives of General Psychiatry, 28*, 111–116.

Eisler, R. M., Hersen, M., & Agras, W. S. (1973). Effects of videotape and instructional feedback on nonverbal marital interaction: An analog study. *Behaviour Therapy, 4*, 551–558.

Eisler, R. M., Miller, P. M., Hersen, M., & Alford, H. (1974). Effects of Assertive Training on marital interaction. *Archives of General Psychiatry, 30*, 643–649.

Falloon, I. R. H. (Ed.). (1988). *Handbook of behavioral family therapy*. New York: Guilford.

Falloon, I. R. H., Boyd, J. L., & McGill, C. W. (1984). *Family care of schizophrenia*. New York: Guilford.

Falloon, I. R. H., Hole, V., Pembleton, T., & Norris, L. J. (1988). Behavioral family interventions in the management of manic-depressive disorders. In J. F. Clarkin, G. Haas, & I. D. Glick (Eds.), *Family intervention in affective illness*. New York: Guilford.

Falloon, I. R. H., & Liberman, R. P. (1983). Behavioral family interventions in the management of chronic schizophrenia. In W. McFarlane (Ed.), *Family therapy of schizophrenia* (pp. 117–140). New York: Guilford.

Falloon, I. R. H., Liberman, R. P., Lillie, F., & Vaughn, C. E. (1981). Family therapy with schizophrenics at high risk of relapse. *Family Process, 20*, 211–221.

Gottman, J., Notarius, C., Gonso, J., & Markman, H. (1976). *A couples guide to communication*. Champaign, IL: Research Press.

Jacobson, N. S. (1985). A component analysis of behavioral marital therapy. *Journal of Consulting and Clinical Psychology, 52*, 295–305.

Jacobson, N. S., & Margolin, G. (1979). *Marital therapy: Strategies based on social learning and behavior exchange principles*. New York: Brunner/Mazel.

Liberman, R. P. (1972). Behavioral methods in group and family therapy. *Seminars in Psychiatry, 4*, 145–156.

Liberman, R. P., Cardin, V. A., McGill, C. W., Falloon, I. R. H., & Evans, C. (1987). Behavioral family management of schizophrenia: Clinical outcomes and costs. *Psychiatric Annals, 17*, 610–619.

Liberman, R. P., & Falloon, I. R. H. (1984). Multiple family therapy for schizophrenia: A behavioral problem-solving approach. *Psychosocial Rehabilitation Journal, 7*, 60–72.

Liberman, R. P., Wallace, C. J., Vaughn, C. E., Snyder, K. S., & Rust, C. (1980). Social and family factors in the course of schizophrenia: Toward an interpersonal problem-solving therapy for schizophrenics and their families. In J. Strauss, S. Flec, & M. Bowers (Eds.), *Psychotherapy of schizophrenia* (pp. 21–54). New York: Plenum.

Liberman, R. P., Wheeler, E., DeVisser, L., Kuehnel, J., & Kuehnel, T. G. (1980). *Handbook of marital therapy*. New York: Plenum.

Liberman, R. P., Wheeler, E., DeVisser, L., Kuehnel, J., & Kuehnel, T. (1983). *Handbook of marital therapy*. New York: Plenum.

Margolin, G. (1983). An interactional model for the behavioral assessment of marital relationships. *Behavioral Assessment, 5*, 103–127.

Margolin, G., & Weiss, R. L. (1978). Communication training and assessment: A case of behavioral marital enrichment. *Behavior Therapy, 9*, 508–520.

Miller, S., Wackman, D. B., & Nunnally, E. W. (1982). *Communication skills for couples*. Minneapolis: Interpersonal Communication Programs.

Patterson, G. R., Hops, H., & Weiss, R. (1975). Interpersonal skills training for couples in early stages of conflict. *Journal of Marriage and Family Counseling, 37*, 295–303.

Stuart, R. B. (1980). *Helping couples change: A social learning approach to marital therapy.* New York: Guilford.

Wampler, K. S. (1982). The effectiveness of the Minnesota Couple Communication program: A review of research. *Journal of Marital and Family Therapy, 8,* 245–256.

Weiss, R. L. (1980). Strategic behavioral marital therapy: Toward a model for assessment and intervention. In J. P. Vincent (Ed.), *Advances in family intervention, assessment and theory: An annual compilation of research* (Vol. 1). Greenwich, CT: JAI Press.

Friendship and Dating

Azrin, R. D., & Hayes, S. C. (1984). The discrimination of interest within a heterosexual interaction: Training, generalization, and effects on social skills. *Behavior Therapy, 15,* 173–184.

Bander, K. W., Steinke, G. V., Allen, G. J., & Mosher, D. L. (1975). Evaluation of three dating-specific treatment approaches for heterosexual dating anxiety. *Journal of Consulting and Clinical Psychology, 43,* 259–265.

Barlow, D. H., Abel, G. G., Blanchard, E. B., Bristow, A. R., & Young, L. D. (1979). A heterosocial skills behavior checklist for males. *Behavior Therapy, 8,* 229–239.

Clark, K. A., Christoff, K. A., & Hansen, D. J. (1986). Friendship-making training for psychiatric aftercare clients. *Journal of Partial Hospitalization, 3,* 273–284.

Conger, J. C., & Conger, A. J. (1982). Components of heterosocial competence. In J. P. Curran & P. M. Monti (Eds.), *Social skills training: A practical handbook for assessment and treatment.* New York: Guilford.

Curran, J. P. (1977). Skills training as an approach to the treatment of heterosexual-social anxiety: A review. *Psychological Bulletin, 84,* 140–157.

Foxx, R. M., McMorrow, M. J., & Schloss, C. N. (1983). Stacking the deck: Teaching social skills to retarded adults with a modified table game. *Journal of Applied Behavior Analysis, 16,* 157–170.

Foxx, R. M., McMorrow, M. J., Storey, K., & Rogers, B. M. (1984). Teaching social/sexual skills to mentally retarded adults. *American Journal of Mental Deficiency, 89,* 9–15.

Kelly, J. A., Urey, J. R., & Patterson, J. T. (1980). Improving heterosocial conversational skills of male psychiatric patients through a small group training procedure. *Behavior Therapy, 11,* 179–188.

Kupke, T. E., Calhoun, K. S., & Hobbs, S. (1979). Selection of heterosocial skills. II. Experimental validity. *Behavior Therapy, 10,* 336–346.

Kupke, T. E., Hobbs, S. A., & Cheney, T. H. (1979). Selection of heterosocial skills. I. Criterion-related validity. *Behavior Therapy, 10,* 323–336.

Lindquist, C. W., Framer, J. A., McGrath, R. A., MacDonald, M. L., & Rhyne, L. D. (1975). Social skills training: Dating skills treatment manual. *JSAS Catalog of Selected Documents in Psychology, 5,* 279.

Lukoff, D., Gioia-Hasick, D., Sullivan, G., Golden, J. S., & Nuechterlein, K. H. (1986). Sex education and rehabilitation with schizophrenic male outpatients. *Schizophrenia Bulletin, 12,* 669–677.

McGovern, K. B., Arkowitz, H., & Gilmore, S. K. (1975). Evaluation of social skills training programs for college dating inhibitions. *Journal of Consulting Psychology, 22,* 505–512.

Muehlenhard, C. L., Koralewski, M. A., Andrews, S. L., Burdick, C. A. (1986). Verbal cues that convey interest in dating: Two studies. *Behavior Therapy, 17,* 404–419.

Mueser, K. T., Valenti-Hein, D., & Yarnold, P. R. (1987). Dating skills groups for the developmentally disabled. *Behavior Modification, 11,* 200–228.

Juvenile Delinquency

DeLange, J. M., Lanham, S. L., & Barton, J. A. (1981). Social skills training for juvenile delinquents: Behavioral skill training and cognitive techniques. In D. Upper & S. M. Ross (Eds.), *Behavioral group therapy: An annual review.* Champaign, IL: Research Press.

Freedman, B. J., Rosenthal, L., Donahoe, C. P., Schlundt, D. G., & McFall, R. M. (1978). A social-behavioral analysis of skills deficits in delinquent and non-delinquent adolescent boys. *Journal of Consulting and Clinical Psychology, 46,* 1448–1462.

Gaffrey, L. F., & McFall, R. M. (1981). A comparison of social skills in delinquent and nondelinquent adolescent girls using a behavioral roleplaying inventory. *Journal of Consulting and Clinical Psychology, 49,* 959–967.

Kifer, R. E., Lewis, M. A., Green, D. R., & Phillips, E. L. (1974). Training pre-delinquent youths and their parents to negotiate conflict situations. *Journal of Applied Behavior Analysis, 7,* 357–364.

Kirigin, K. A., Wolf, M., Braukman, C. J., Fixsen, D. L., & Phillips, E. L. (1979). Achievement place outcome evaluation. In J. S. Stumphauzer (Ed.), *Progress in behavior therapy with delinquents.* Springfield, IL: C. C. Thomas.

Ollendick, T. H., & Hersen, M. (1979). Social skills training for juvenile delinquents. *Behavior Research and Therapy, 17,* 547–554.

Phillips, E. L., Phillips, E. A., Fixsen, D. A., & Wolf, M. M. (1974). *The teaching family handbook.* Lawrence: University of Kansas Printing Service.

Spence, S. H. (1979). Social skills training with adolescent offenders: A review. *Behavioral Psychotherapy, 7,* 49–56.

Spence, S. (1982). Social skills training with young offenders. In P. Feldman (Ed.), *Developments in the study of criminal behaviour: Vol. 1. The prevention and control of offending.* Chichester: John Wiley.

Spence, S. (1983). Adolescent offenders in an institutional setting. Social skills training with adolescent male offenders: I. Short-term effects. *Behaviour Research and Therapy, 17,* 7–16.

Problem Solving

Bedell, J. R., Archer, R. P., & Marlowe, H. A., Jr. (1980). A description and evaluation of a problem-solving skills training program. In D. Upper & S. M. Ross (Eds.), *Behavioral group therapy: An annual review.* Champaign, IL: Research Press.

Bellack, A. S., Morrison, R. L., & Mueser, K. T. (in press). Social problem solving in schizophrenia. *Schizophrenia Bulletin.*

Castles, E. E., & Glass, C. R. (1986). Training in social and interpersonal problem-solving skills for mildly and moderately retarded adults. *American Journal of Mental Deficiency, 91,* 35–42.

Cormier, W. H., Otani, A., & Cormier, L. S. (1986). The effects of problem-solving training on two problem-solving tasks. *Cognitive Therapy and Research, 19,* 95–108.

D'Zurilla, T. J. (1986). *Problem-solving therapy.* New York: Springer.

D'Zurilla, T. J., & Goldfried, M. R. (1971). Problem solving and behavior modification. *Journal of Abnormal Psychology, 78,* 107–126.

Edelstein, B. A., Couture, E., Cray, D. M., Dicken, P., & Lusebrink, N. (1980). Group training of problem solving with psychiatric patients. In D. Upper & S. M. Ross (Eds.), *Behavioral group therapy: An annual review.* Champaign, IL: Research Press.

Hains, A. A. (1984). A preliminary attempt to teach the use of social problem-solving skills to delinquents. *Child Study Journal, 14,* 271–285.

Hansen, D. J., St. Lawrence, J. S., and Christoff, K. A. (1985). Effects of interpersonal problem-solving training with chronic aftercare patients on problem-solving component skills and effectiveness of solutions. *Journal of Consulting and Clinical Psychology, 53,* 167–174.

Kagen, C. (1984). Social problem-solving and social skills training. *British Journal of Clinical Psychology, 23,* 161–173.

Kalfus, G. R., Hawkins, R. P., & Reitz, A. L. (1984). A program for teaching problem solving in a school for disturbed-delinquent adolescent youth. *Journal of Child Development and Adolescent Psychotherapy, 1,* 26–29.

Siegel, J. M., & Spivack, G. (1976). Problem-solving therapy: The description of a new program for chronic psychiatric patients. *Psychotherapy: Theory, Research and Practice, 13,* 368–373.

Social Perception

Feinberg, T. E., Rifkin, A., Schzifer, C., & Walker, E. (1986). Facial discrimination and emotion recognition in schizophrenia and affective disorders. *Archives of General Psychiatry, 43,* 276–279.

Fingeret, A. L., Monti, P. M., & Paxson, M. A. (1985). Social perception, social performance, and self-perception. *Behavior Modification, 9,* 345–356.

Morrison, R. L., & Bellack, A. S. (1981). The role of social perception in social skill. *Behavior Therapy, 12,* 69–79.

Morrison, R. L., Bellack, A. S., & Mueser, K. T. (in press). Facial affect recognition deficits and schizophrenia. *Schizophrenia Bulletin.*

Vocational Skills

Argyle, M. (Ed.). *Social skills and work.* London: Methuen.

Black, J. L., Muehlenhard, C. L., & Massey, F. H. (1985). Social skills training to improve job maintenance. *Journal of Employment Counseling, 22,* 151–160.

Calabrese, D. N., & Hawkins, R. P. (1988). Job-related social skills training with female prisoners. *Behavior Modification, 12,* 3–34.

Eagan, I., Fredericks, H. B., & Hendrickson, K. (1985). Teaching associated work skills to adolescents with severe handicaps. *Education and Treatment of Children, 8,* 239–250.

Eisler, R. M. (1976). Assertive Training in the work situation. In J. D. Krumboltz & C. E. Thoresen (Eds.), *Behavioral counseling methods.* New York: Holt, Rinehart and Winston.

Foy, D. W., Massey, F. H., Duer, J. D., Ross, J. M., & Wooten, L. S. (1979). Social skills training to improve alcoholics vocational interpersonal competency. *Journal of Counseling Psychology, 26,* 128–132.

Furman, W., Geller, M., Simon, S. J., & Kelly, J. A. (1979). The use of a behavioral rehearsal procedure for teaching job interview skills to psychiatric patients. *Behavior Therapy, 10,* 157–167.

Heimberg, R. G., Cunningham, J., Heimberg, J. S., & Blankenberg, R. (1982). Preparing unemployed youth for job interviews: A controlled evaluation. *Behavior Modification, 6,* 299–322.

Hollandsworth, J. G., Jr., Glazeski, R. C., & Dressel, M. E. (1978). Use of social skills training in the treatment of extreme anxiety and deficient verbal skills in the job-interview setting. *Journal of Applied Behavior Analysis, 11,* 259–269.

Hood, E., Lindsay, W., & Brooks, N. (1982). Interview training with adolescents—a controlled group study incorporating generalization and social validation. *Behaviour Research and Therapy, 20,* 581–592.

Jacobs, H. E., Kardashian, S., Kreinbring, R. K., Ponder, R., & Simpson, A. R. (1984). A skills-oriented model for facilitating employment among psychiatrically disabled persons. *Rehabilitation Counseling Bulletin, 28,* 87–96.

Kelly, J. A., & Christoff, K. A. (1985). Job interview training. *Psychiatric Aspects of Mental Retardation Reviews, 4,* 5–8.

Kelly, J. A., Laughlin, C., Claiborne, M., & Patterson, J. (1979). A group procedure for teaching job interviewing skills to formerly hospitalized psychiatric patients. *Behavior Therapy, 10,* 79–83.

Kiel, E. C., & Barbee, J. R. (1973). Training the disadvantaged job interviewee. *Vocational Guidance Quarterly, 22,* 50–56.

Mueser, K. T., Foy, D. W., & Carter, M. J. (1986). Social skills training for job maintenance in a psychiatric patient. *Journal of Counseling Psychology, 33,* 360–362.

Mueser, K. T., & Liberman, R. P. (1988). Vocational skills training. In J. A. Ciardello & M. D. Bell (Eds.), *Vocational rehabilitation of persons with prolonged mental illness.* Baltimore: Johns Hopkins University Press.

Vernardoes, M. H., & Harris, M. B. (1973). Job interview training with rehabilitation clients. *Journal of Applied Psychology, 58,* 365–367.

Training Therapists to Conduct Social Skills Training

Anthony, W. A. (1979). *Principles of psychiatric rehabilitation and skills training procedures.* Baltimore: University Park Press.

Goldstein, A. P., & Goedhart, A. (1973). The use of structured learning for empathy enhancement in paraprofessional psychotherapist training. *Journal of Community Psychology, 1,* 168–173.

Liberman, R. P., & Bryan, E. (1977). Behavior therapy in a community mental health center. *American Journal of Psychiatry, 134,* 401–406.

Liberman, R. P., Eckman, T., Kuehnel, T., Rosenstein, J., & Kuehnel, J. (1982). Dissemination of new behavior therapy programs to community mental health centers. *American Journal of Psychiatry, 139,* 224–226.

Munford, P., Alevizos, P., Miller, W. H., Callahan, E. J., Liberman, R. P., & Guilani, B. (1979). A behavioral approach to behavior therapy training. *Journal of Psychiatric Education, 4,* 47–51.

Psychiatric Rehabilitation Consultants. Manuals, Resource Books, and Training Videos. (Available from Dissemination Coordinator, Camarillo-UCLA Research Center, Box A, Camarillo, CA 93011)

Rogers, E. S., Cohen, B. F., Danley, K. S., Hutchinson, D., & Anthony, W. A. (1986). Training mental health workers in psychiatric rehabilitation. *Schizophrenia Bulletin, 12,* 709–719.

Author Index

Subject Index

About the Authors

Robert Paul Liberman, M.D., is Professor of Psychiatry at the UCLA School of Medicine where he directs the Clinical Research Center for Schizophrenia & Psychiatric Rehabilitation. He is concurrently Chief of the Rehabilitation Service of the Brentwood (Psychiatric) Division of the West Los Angeles VA Medical Center which serves as a national demonstration site for innovation in social and independent living skills and vocational rehabilitation of the chronic mentally ill. Liberman has directed the Clinical Research Unit at Camarillo State Hospital, which is the longest lived behavior therapy unit in the world, since 1970. Liberman has received awards from the American Psychiatric Association, the American Academy of Psychoanalysis and the California Alliance for the Mentally Ill. His research on stress-vulnerability-coping-competence in schizophrenia has led to the design and worldwide dissemination of effective modalities for treatment and rehabilitation.

William J. DeRisi, Ph.D., is Chief of the Program Development and Evaluation Branch of the California Department of Mental Health where he has enhanced psychosocial treatment of the seriously mentally ill in state hospitals through instituting a program of planned and scheduled therapies. He has directed research and development projects in facilities for juvenile delinquents and community mental health and is co-author of the best-selling book, *Writing Behavioral Contracts*. He received his doctorate in psychology from the University of Utah.

Kim T. Mueser, Ph.D., is Assistant Professor of Psychiatry at the Medical College of Pennsylvania, where he coordinates the Schizophrenia Treatment Program at Eastern Pennsylvania Psychiatric Institute. Mueser conducts clinical research on the role of social skills and social competence as protective factors in schizophrenia and maintains the fidelity of family skills training in a collaborative, multisite study of innovative drug and psychosocial therapies for schizophrenics. He has authored over 50 journal articles and book chapters on topics such as behavioral assessment, social skills training, behavioral family therapy, and psychosocial treatment of severe psychiatric illness. He recently received a Fellowship Award from the National Alliance for Research in Schizophrenia and Affective Disorders to study the effects of social skills training with psychiatric inpatients. He received his doctorate in psychology from the University of Illinois at Chicago.

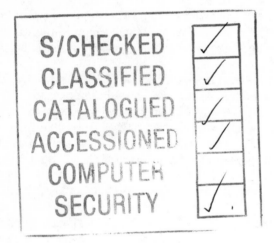